T0177915

REGIONAL
ANAESTHESIA

A POCKET GUIDE

REGIONAL ANAESTHESIA

A POCKET GUIDE

DR ALWIN CHUAN

&

DR DAVID M SCOTT

OXFORD
UNIVERSITY PRESS

OXFORD
UNIVERSITY PRESS

Great Clarendon Street, Oxford, OX2 6DP,
United Kingdom

Oxford University Press is a department of the University of Oxford.
It furthers the University's objective of excellence in research, scholarship,
and education by publishing worldwide. Oxford is a registered trade mark of
Oxford University Press in the UK and in certain other countries

Published in the United States of America by Oxford University Press
198 Madison Avenue, New York, NY 10016, United States of America

British Library Cataloguing in Publication Data
Data available

Library of Congress Control Number: 2013955153

ISBN 978-0-19-968423-6

Printed in Great Britain by
Ashford Colour Press Ltd, Gosport, Hampshire

CONTENTS

ABBREVIATIONS

a.	artery
ASIS	anterior superior iliac spine
CFD	colour flow Doppler
cm	centimetre
CNS	central nervous system
CPR	cardiopulmonary resuscitation
2D	two-dimensional
ECG	electrocardiogram
h	hour
IP	in-plane
IT	ischial tuberosity
kg	kilogram
L	litre
LA	local anaesthetic
LAX	long axis
m.	muscle
mA	milliampere
MHz	megahertz
min	minute
mL	millilitre
mm	millimetre
mm.	muscles
mmHg	millimetre of mercury
ms	millisecond
n.	nerve
NSAID	non-steroidal anti-inflammatory drug
OOP	out-of-plane
PSIS	posterior superior iliac spine
SAX	short axis
scm	sternocleidomastoid
TAP	transversus abdominis plane
U	unit
v.	vein

PREFACE

Regional anaesthesia is an essential component of the anaesthetists' skill set. Correct application of regional anaesthesia provides opportunity for enhanced patient recovery and rehabilitation through improved perioperative analgesia and reduced doses of systemic anaesthetic and analgesic agents.

Successful regional anaesthesia relies on two critical tasks: the identification of target nerves within their anatomical surroundings and the application of local anaesthetic solution as close as possible to the target nerve.

First published in Australia, the *Regional Anaesthesia Pocket Guide* was written as a quick-reference pocketbook, full of clinical photographs and anatomical drawings, to help anaesthetists apply anatomical knowledge in practical anaesthetic procedures. Following on from its success amongst consultants and trainees, the authors have revised the text to reflect the evolving practice of ultrasound guidance in anaesthesia practice and given the book a more international focus. High-frequency ultrasound allows better visualization of target nerves and identification of individual anatomical variation. Real-time observation of needle placement permits more accurate deposition of local anaesthetic solution, reducing the total volume and dose required and reducing the risk of inadvertent puncture of blood vessels and other vulnerable structures.

This new international edition of *Regional Anaesthesia* places added emphasis on ultrasound-guided blocks; suitable landmark-based blocks have been retained for practitioners who do not have access to ultrasound guidance. Blocks where ultrasound guidance is not relevant, such as blocks of the head, are also included.

We are confident that this unique compilation of regional anaesthesia techniques for peripheral and para-axial nerve blocks will continue to support the application of regional anaesthesia within your anaesthetic practice.

Alwin Chuan and David Scott

ABOUT THE AUTHORS

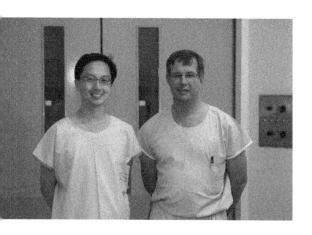

Dr Alwin Chuan MB BS (Hons), PGCertCU, FANZCA,
Consultant Anaesthetist, Sydney, New South Wales

Dr Chuan has a strong interest in perioperative ultrasonography, including ultrasound-guided regional anaesthesia. He has been a guest speaker and workshop tutor in Australia and internationally and has written on ultrasound-guided regional techniques. Dr Chuan is actively involved in curriculum development of the postgraduate ultrasound degrees at the University of Melbourne and in the Regional Anaesthesia Special Interest Group of the ASA/ANZCA/NZSA. Dr Chuan is a VMO at Liverpool Hospital, Sydney, where he helped to establish an Anaesthesia Fellowship in perioperative ultrasonography.

Dr David M Scott BMed, PGCertCU, FANZCA,
Consultant Anaesthetist, Lismore Base Hospital,
Lismore, New South Wales

Dr Scott has interests in regional anaesthesia and military anaesthesia. Dr Scott is the founding chairman of the Regional Anaesthesia Special Interest Group of the ASA/ANZCA/NZSA. He has lectured on regional anaesthesia extensively, nationally and internationally, and has facilitated many regional anaesthesia workshops. Dr Scott is also a Group Captain in the Royal Australian Air Force Specialist Reserve and has been deployed overseas on many missions.

CHAPTER ONE

INTRODUCTION TO REGIONAL ANAESTHESIA

Pre-anaesthesia

Patient consultation prior to anaesthesia[1]

- Anaesthetists should consult with patients prior to scheduled anaesthesia to assess the patient's medical status and plan appropriate anaesthesia management:
  - Introduce themselves to the patient
  - Complete an appropriate medical assessment of the patient
  - Discuss details of the anaesthetic management that may be of significance to the patient, including complications of regional anaesthesia techniques
  - Obtain informed consent for the anaesthesia and related procedures
  - Order medications considered necessary
  - Consult with professional colleagues, if required
  - Document a summary of the consultation.

Equipment and operation room

- Resuscitation equipment and drugs should be readily available and easily accessible in the room that the regional anaesthesia procedure is performed
- In Australia and New Zealand, refer to Australian and New Zealand College of Anaesthetists Professional Document T1 'Recommendations on minimum facilities for safe administration of anaesthesia in operating suites and other anaesthetising locations' (http://www.anzca.edu.au/resources/professional-documents/technical/t1.html).

Examples of regional anaesthesia needles and catheters

Examples of regional anaesthesia needles and catheters can be seen in Box 1.1.

Nerve stimulators

- Detailed descriptions of the requirements for, and use of, nerve stimulators can be found at the New York School of Regional Anaesthesia website (http://www.nysora.com/regional_ anaesthesia/equipment/3114-nerve_stimulators.html).

BOX 1.1 REGIONAL ANAESTHESIA NEEDLES AND CATHETERS

Single shot
- Stimuplex® (B. Braun)
  - A series: 30° bevel
  - D series: 15° or 30° bevel.
- UniPlex (PAJUNK®)
  - SPROTTE® or Tuohy cannulae.

Continuous
- StimuCath™ (Arrow)
- Contiplex® (B. Braun)
- Plexolong (PAJUNK®)
  - SPROTTE®, Tuohy, or Facet cannulae.
- Stimulong Plus (PAJUNK®)
  - Direct stimulation of the nerve by the catheter.

Spinal needle
- Spinocan® (B. Braun)
  - Quincke bevel
- Spinocath® (B. Braun)
  - Continuous injection
- SPROTTE® Pencil Point Spinal Needle (B. Braun).
- Whitacre Pencil Point Spinal Needle (BD)
- Gertie Marx® Spinal Needle (IMD).

General technical guidelines for performing regional anaesthesia

- Ensure technique is aseptic for epidural and spinal blocks, and for major peripheral nerve blocks
- Prior to performing the nerve block, infiltrate the needle insertion site with local anaesthetic:
  - If available and time permits, pre-treat the injection site with a topical local anaesthetic cream to lessen the pain of injection. Most studies investigating the supplementation of topical analgesia with infiltration anaesthesia demonstrated reduced pain experienced during infiltration[2]
- If using a short bevel needle (e.g. 45° bevel), it may be useful to incise the skin with a lancet before needle insertion
- When using nerve stimulation:
  - Stimulate nerves at 1.0 mA until muscle contractions are visible in the corresponding innervation area. Reduce current to between 0.3 mA/0.1 ms and 0.5 mA/0.1 ms before injecting the local anaesthetic
  - An immediate loss of muscle response with injection of 0.5 mL saline or local anaesthetic (Raj test) is reassuring. Alternatively, inject 1 mL 5% dextrose, which maintains or augments the motor response, followed by local anaesthetic[3]
- When injecting large doses of local anaesthetic, inject in fractions and maintain verbal communication with the patient for early detection of accidental intravascular injection. Avoid forceful injection
- In patients who are uncooperative or under sedation, or when performing a block distal to an established central block (e.g. femoral nerve block in the presence of spinal anaesthesia), use a nerve stimulator and an insulated needle (but not for infiltration anaesthesia of purely sensory nerves) or ultrasound
- Monitor patients:
  - Clinical monitoring of fundamental physiological variables is essential. Monitor the patient's cardiorespiratory status at frequent and clinically appropriate intervals, and interpret the patient's oximetric values in conjunction with clinical observation. Standard monitoring equipment includes a pulse oximeter, ECG, temperature monitor, and frequent blood pressure measurement.[4]

Catheter technique for continuous infusions

Preparation

- Perform continuous infusions using a sterile technique, with gown and gloves, as for placement of an epidural
- Prepare skin appropriately. If using alcohol-containing solutions, take care to avoid contamination of the catheter with the solution, as it is neurotoxic and may move along the catheter by capillary action
- Drape the field appropriately.

Continuous catheter technique

- Unless otherwise specified, direct and place the needle as described for the single injection technique. With ultrasound, it may be helpful to use a slightly oblique approach for in-plane needle visualization
- Confirm needle placement by stimulation of appropriate muscles if using a nerve stimulator
- If using a stimulating catheter, e.g. StimuCath™:
  - Advance the catheter through the needle, and attach the stimulator to the catheter
  - Advance the catheter while stimulating (a higher stimulating current may be required)
  - If muscle twitch is lost, withdraw the catheter; rotate the needle slightly; reattain muscle twitch, then readvance the catheter
  - Confirm catheter position, and withdraw the needle, leaving the catheter in place
  - Tunnel the catheter, if desired
  - Inject initial bolus of local anaesthetic through the catheter while stimulating—muscle twitch should be immediately abolished
- If using a non-stimulating catheter, e.g. Plexolong or Contiplex® (19.5 G, insulated Tuohy needle and 20 G catheter):
  - Inject a small bolus of local anaesthetic or saline—this creates a space for the catheter to be placed
  - Pass the catheter firmly, but not forcefully, through the needle until it is 2–5 cm beyond the needle tip, visualizing with ultrasound, if available
  - Remove the needle, taking care not to dislodge the catheter
  - If the catheter has an internal wire, it should be removed at this point
- Inject local anaesthetic for surgical anaesthesia through catheter while visualizing with ultrasound, if available
- Secure the catheter with an adhesive dressing, and consider subcutaneous tunnelling
- Infuse local anaesthetic at a rate of 2–10 mL/h
- Alternatively, a patient-controlled regional anaesthesia pump can be programmed for a 2 mL/h infusion and 5 mL bolus with 30-minute lockout.

Ultrasound-guided regional anaesthesia

Ultrasound-guided regional anaesthesia allows identification and visualization of:[5-8]

- Neural structures and their relationship to anatomical planes
- Surrounding critical structures, such as pleura and blood vessels
- Anatomical variations in individual patients
- The needle tip
- The spread of local anaesthetic around the target structures.

Visualization of the nerve's anatomical relationships and the needle tip position may allow:[5-8]

- Optimal positioning of the needle
- Minimization of potential complications, such as intravascular and intraneural injection, and tissue damage
- Re-insertion or redirection of the needle to accommodate for anatomical variation
- Real-time repositioning of the needle during blockade if the local anaesthetic spreads in the wrong direction and does not surround the nerve.

Potential advantages of ultrasound-guided regional anaesthesia include:[5-8]

- Reduced reliance on surface anatomy landmarks for needle insertion, particularly in the trauma, post-surgical, congenital deformity, or morbidly obese patient populations
- Decrease in local anaesthetic dose required for an effective block
- Faster sensory onset times
- Longer duration of blocks
- Improved quality of block.

Equipment

Ultrasound machine

See Figure 1.1.

Linear-array ultrasound probes (>10 MHz)

High frequency provides excellent resolution of peripheral nerves. However, deeper nerves are less well visualized, as penetration is reduced. The large transducer face allows for a wider field of view but can make it difficult to maintain skin contact in paediatric patients and patients with a smaller body habitus. See Figure 1.2.

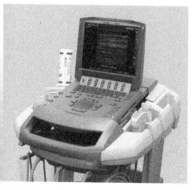

FIGURE 1.1 Ultrasound machine.

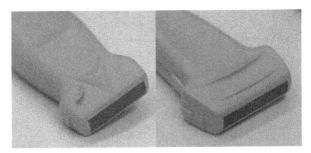

FIGURE 1.2 Linear-array ultrasound probes.

Curvilinear ultrasound probes (2–5 MHz)

These provide better penetration than linear array probes and are useful when visualizing deeper nerves, such as the lumbar plexus. The transducer face is larger than that of linear probes and allows for a wide field of view. See Figure 1.3.

Ultrasound spatial terms

Figures 1.4 and 1.5 demonstrate ultrasound spatial terms.

First-principles approach to ultrasound-guided blocks

Scanning technique

- In the SAX view (see Figure 1.6), with the probe perpendicular to the long axis of the nerve, the nerve appears in a round to oval shape, with internal hypoechoic nerve fascicles surrounded by the hyperechoic epineurium[9]
- In the LAX view (see Figure 1.7), the nerve appears as a linear hypoechoic fascicular component mixed with hyperechoic bands which correspond to the interfascicular epineurium.[9]

Appearance of nerves and blood vessels with ultrasound

- Several factors may influence the appearance of nerves when imaged using ultrasound:
  - Ultrasound resolution
  - Imaging depth
  - Nerve structure
  - Probe angle

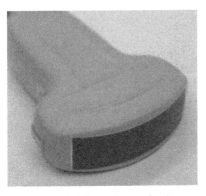

FIGURE 1.3 Curvilinear ultrasound probe.

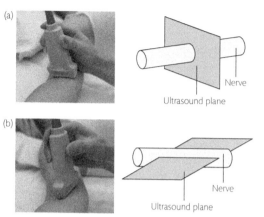

FIGURE 1.4 Nerve views. (a) Short axis (SAX) view. The ultrasound imaging plane is perpendicular to the nerve. (b) Long axis (LAX) view. The ultrasound imaging plane is parallel to the nerve.

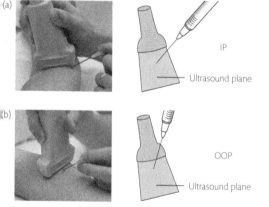

FIGURE 1.5 Needle approach. (a) In-plane (IP) approach. The needle is imaged along the entirety of its shaft within the ultrasound plane. (b) Out-of-plane (OOP) approach. The needle is inserted at right angles to the imaging plane. Move the imaging plane to keep the needle tip in constant view as the needle is advanced.

- The characteristic appearance of nerves at various locations may assist in their identification. Lower frequencies increase the penetration of ultrasound energy—useful for the identification of deeper nerves—at the expense of resolution
- The neck is the only location where it is possible to image nerve roots and the proximal few centimetres of peripheral nerves, visible as a dark centre surrounded by a hyperechoic rim
- The appearance of peripheral nerves in cross section may vary from rounded to flattened

(a)

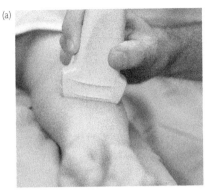

(b)

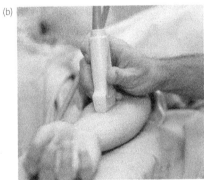

FIGURE 1.6 (a) SAX view of the median nerve forearm. (b) LAX view of the median nerve forearm.

- Anisotropy is a helpful property for the identification of peripheral nerves. It is recognized as the enhanced ultrasound reflection when the nerve is imaged perpendicular to the fibre direction. See Figures 1.8 and 1.9
  - Tendons share a similar characteristic and must be differentiated from nerves prior to nerve blockade. Tendons disappear into muscles when scanned proximally. See Figure 1.10
- The echogenicity of nerves varies, according to their location. Peripheral branches of the sciatic nerve and brachial plexus, for example, are predominantly hyperechoic, while nerve roots and trunks of the brachial plexus in the interscalene and supraclavicular region appear hypoechoic.[9] See Figures 1.11 and 1.12
- Blood vessels are frequently used as landmarks for the localization of nerves:
  - Well-demarcated vessel walls surround the sonolucent black blood flow
  - Arteries are rounder, with thick walls, and may be pulsatile
  - Veins have thinner, readily collapsible walls when gentle pressure is applied
  - Colour flow Doppler and colour power Doppler may assist with the identification of vessels. See Figures 1.13 and 1.14
  - Vessels usually have a post-cystic enhancement.

(a)

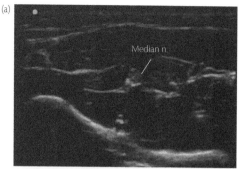

(b)

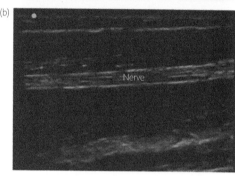

FIGURE 1.7 (a) SAX view of the median nerve. (b) LAX view of the median nerve.

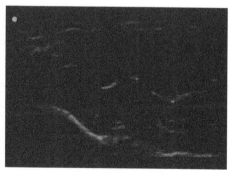

FIGURE 1.8 Anisotropy (median nerve not visible).

Preoperative assessment

- Routine preoperative assessment is still required prior to performing ultrasound-guided blocks
- Remember to consider contraindications
- Informed consent is required prior to performing ultrasound-guided blocks; specific information should be provided to patients:
  - Example forms are available at: (http://www.acecc.org.au/default.aspx)
  - Refer to resources under the Regional Anaesthesia Special Interest Group (SIG) (http://www.acecc.org.au/RegAnaes.aspx).

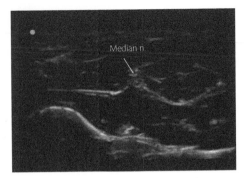

FIGURE 1.9 Anisotropy (median nerve visible).

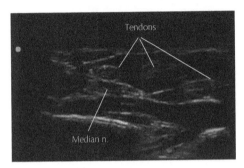

FIGURE 1.10 Median nerve and tendons.

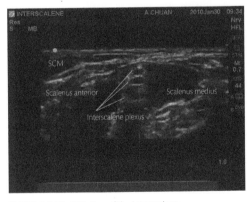

FIGURE 1.11 SAX view of the interscalene.

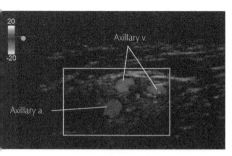

FIGURE 1.12 SAX view of the axillary uncompressed CFD.

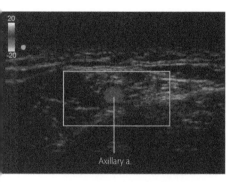

FIGURE 1.13 SAX view of the axillary compressed CFD.

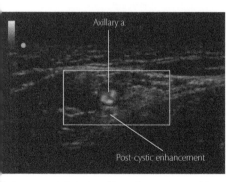

FIGURE 1.14 SAX view of the axillary compressed CFD.

Set-up and equipment

- Optimal ergonomics are essential for the success of ultrasound-guided regional anaesthesia:[10]
  - The patient is positioned appropriately for the specific block to be administered
  - The operator should ensure that the ultrasound screen is easily seen without the need to twist or turn their body—this may be on the opposite side of the patient
  - Figures 1.15 and 1.16 demonstrate good and bad ergonomics for ultrasound-guided regional anaesthesia

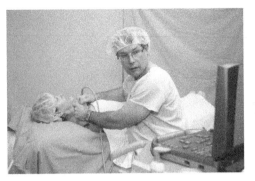

FIGURE 1.15 Bad ergonomics for ultrasound-guided regional anaesthesia.

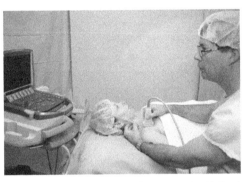

FIGURE 1.16 Good ergonomics for ultrasound-guided regional anaesthesia.

- Ensure all equipment is prepared prior to application of the probe so that the block procedure may continue immediately without the need to reorientate:[10]
  - The ultrasound probe should be covered with a sterile plastic sheath, ensuring no seam overlies the tip
  - Depending on the type of probe, water, saline, or gel may be used inside the sheath, and sterile gel, water, saline, or antiseptic solution used outside the sheath as a coupling medium between the probe and the patient. Sterile water is recommended when performing central neuraxial block to avoid contact between the needle and ultrasound gel
  - Needle choice will vary with the procedure and the experience of the anaesthetist; larger Tuohy needles are easier for beginners to visualize, while the more experienced may prefer to use finer needles. Echogenic tipped needles are a useful alternative when attempting to block deeper nerves
- Additional personnel should be available to assist the anaesthetist, as required:
  - Non-sterile assistants are required to open sterile items and equipment
  - Sterile/gloved assistants should be available to assist with holding the probe or injection of agents.

Infection control in ultrasound-guided regional anaesthesia

- Published guidelines recommend the use of surgical mask and gloves, following proper handwashing for single shot blocks[11]
- A sterile gown should be added for continuous catheters

- Appropriate infection control practices for the ultrasound machine and probe should be undertaken:
  - Avoid cross-contamination from the probe by sheathing prior to, and decontaminating after, each patient. See Figure 1.17
  - Heavily soiled probes should be cleaned thoroughly with mild detergent.

Preprocedure scanning

- Ultrasonic examination should be performed before deciding on the block:
  - Identify anatomical variations that may preclude specific blocks
  - Optimize ultrasound images
  - Choose procedure, and plan needle path
- The best images are obtained before the probe is in a sterile sheath
- Opportunity to determine the most appropriate block and approach for needle (IP/OOP).

Performing the procedure

Several factors should be considered to maximize the advantages of ultrasound-guided regional anaesthesia.
- Asepsis should be strictly maintained
- Ultrasound-guided regional anaesthesia is not constrained by surface or palpable landmarks. Perform the block at a location such that the projected needle trajectory maximizes needle tip visualization but avoids critical structures to reduce the risk of complications
- Gentle tissue handling skills are required to minimize the risk of iatrogenic damage to anatomical structures:
  - Align the needle trajectory towards the corners of nerves to avoid direct needle trauma if the tip is placed deeper than expected. See Figures 1.18 to 1.21
- Many nerves relevant to regional anaesthesia lie in a fascial plane:
  - Align the needle trajectory towards fascial planes, and hydrodissect the plane with local anaesthesia, saline, or 5% dextrose
  - Correct needle tip placement is confirmed with optimal injectate spread around the nerve. See Figure 1.22

(a)

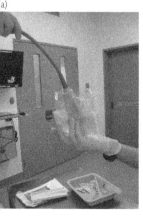

(b)

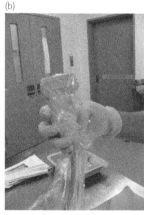

FIGURE 1.17 (a) and (b) Sheathing of probe to prevent cross-contamination.

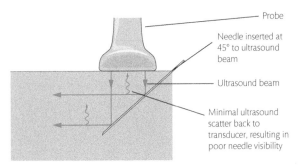

FIGURE 1.18 Needle tip visibilities 45°. The needle is inserted at 45° to the ultrasound probe.

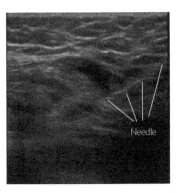

FIGURE 1.19 Needle tip is visible in the ultrasound at 45°.

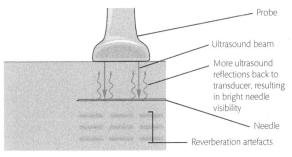

FIGURE 1.20 Needle tip visibilities 90°. Needle is inserted at 90° to ultrasound probe.

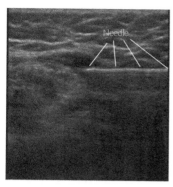

FIGURE 1.21 Needle tip is visible in the ultrasound at 90°.

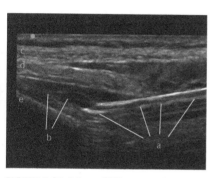

FIGURE 1.22 Subcostal TAP—correct plane.

a	Tuohy needle	c External oblique m.
b	Local anaesthetic hydrodissection in TAP	d Internal oblique m.
		e Transversus abdominis m.

- Needle advancement and injectate spread are best visualized in real time
- Ultrasound-guided regional anaesthesia may be a multi-injection technique, where the needle is repositioned several times to optimize spread of local anaesthetic. Figures 1.23 to 1.26 demonstrate this process of repositioning:
  - Bolus–observe–reposition
- Attention should be paid to the incorporation of ultrasound-guided nerve blocks into the overall flow of the procedure for each patient to allow sufficient time for effective block prior to the procedure and to avoid the block wearing off prematurely.

Troubleshooting for ultrasound-guided regional anaesthesia

- Several steps may be taken if the ultrasound images obtained are of poor quality:[10]
  - Inspect the ultrasound machine settings, including power, frequency, depth, gain, time gain compensation, focus, and software

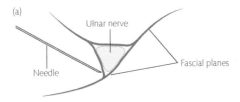

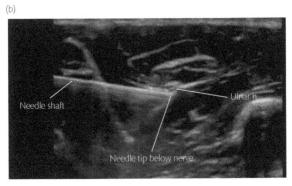

FIGURE 1.23 Ulnar block, step one: aiming for nerve corners. (a) Aim the needle at the corners of the nerves to avoid direct nerve trauma. (b) Correct position of the needle shaft shown in ultrasound.

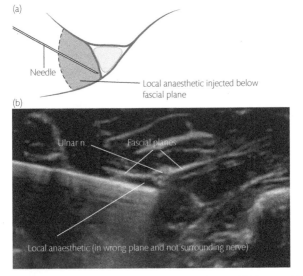

FIGURE 1.24 Ulnar block, step two: bolus and observe. (a) Aim to position needle tip into fascial plane; local anaesthetic will then hydrodissect naturally around nerve target. (b) Here, local anaesthetic is shown in the wrong plane and not surrounding nerve.

(a)

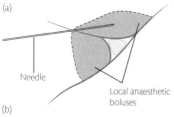

(b)

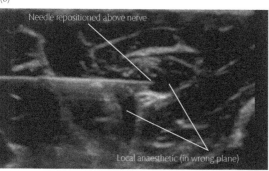

FIGURE 1.25 Ulnar block, step three: reposition, then bolus–observe.
(a) The needle is repositioned above the nerve, aiming at the nerve corner
and into the fascial plane. Bolus demonstrates the position is still incorrect.
(b) The needle has been repositioned but is still in the wrong plane.

(a)

(b)

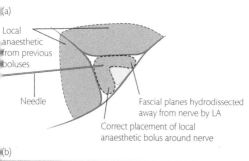

FIGURE 1.26 Ulnar block, step four: ideal placement. (a) The needle is
repositioned again, and another bolus is injected and observed; an ideal
U-shaped spread of local anaesthetic is then observed. (b) The needle is now
shown correctly positioned.

- Ensure sufficient coupling medium exists between the probe and the patient, both within and outside the sheath. Remove any sheath seams or bubbles from over the probe
- Try holding the probe in place, with gentle pressure for a few seconds, to improve the picture quality
- Nerve stimulators may be used in combination with ultrasound to accurately identify individual nerves:[10]
  - Recommended when the operator is unsure of the anatomy
  - Limitations include failure to successfully stimulate the nerve, despite direct contact with the needle, and patient discomfort.

Follow-up

- Follow-up is required to detect any new onset of paraesthesiae, tingling, abnormal sensation, weakness, or pain post-block
- The authors recommend patient follow-up over 7–10 days post-block. A suggested algorithm can be found at the International Registry of Regional Anaesthesia (AURORA), at http://www.anaesthesiaregistry.org.[12]

Troubleshooting for neurostimulation-guided regional anaesthesia

There are many reasons why anaesthetists experience difficulty when performing regional anaesthesia blocks, and it can be difficult to discern why a nerve cannot be located.

If experiencing difficulty, the following tips may be of use:

* Confirm that the nerve stimulator is connected and that the battery is charged
* Ensure the connections are good (wires not broken)
* Ensure good contact with the ECG electrode
* Confirm that an appropriate current is set (start at approximately 1 mA)
* Verify the anatomical landmarks—this is especially important with obese patients. Ensure the correct projection of bony landmarks to the skin, as errors are easily generated when bony landmarks are poorly localized and loose skin causes midline shift
* If the patient is conscious, moving, and uncooperative, consider general anaesthesia prior to regional anaesthesia if the techniques are to be performed together. Evidence suggests that the risk of nerve damage while performing regional anaesthesia blocks is no greater in unconscious patients than in conscious patients
* When learning to perform regional anaesthesia techniques, allow ample time to administer the block and for the block to take effect
* Do not accept an inferior muscle twitch—ensure that the correct muscle is stimulated and that the muscle is not being directly stimulated
* Ensure the stimulating current is low enough to be close to the nerve
* When stimulation achieves the desired muscle twitch, gently inject 0.5 mL of local anaesthetic, which should abolish the twitch. If further stimulation is required, then 5% dextrose should be used as the test bolus. If not, or there is radicular pain or high injection pressures, reposition the needle slightly to avoid intraneural injection
* Always inject local anaesthetic gently, and aspirate gently for every 5 mL of local anaesthetic injected
* Keep the needle immobile while injecting. For blocks where the needle is well held by the tissues (e.g. sciatic nerve block), release of the needle may be advantageous so that, if the patient moves, the needle will remain in position.

General side effects and complications of regional anaesthesia

Systemic toxicity of the local anaesthetic
- Most commonly caused by unintended intravascular injection
- To minimize risk:
  - Adhere to the recommended dosages
  - Aspirate repeatedly, and inject fractionally (negative aspiration does not entirely exclude intravascular injection)
  - Observe spread of local anaesthetic on ultrasound
  - Inject slowly
  - Observe and maintain verbal contact with the patient.

Nerve damage (extremely rare)
- To minimize risk:
  - Ensure needle tip is in view before advancing when using ultrasound
  - Avoid paraesthesiae when inserting the needle
  - Use a suitable nerve stimulator
  - Use atraumatic needles.

Haematoma
- To minimize risk:
  - Consider not performing blocks in patients with a clinically manifest coagulation disorder or receiving anticoagulation treatment
  - Refer to guidelines for regional anaesthesia in patients receiving antithrombotic therapy.[13]

Infection (especially with continuous catheter technique)
- To minimize risk:
  - Insert the needle using an aseptic technique
  - Avoid injection through infected areas
  - Regularly check the catheter insertion site (at least once a day)
  - Immediately remove the catheter if the patient reports tenderness at the point of catheter entry (most sensitive indicator of infection).

General contraindications
See Box 1.2.

BOX 1.2 GENERAL CONTRAINDICATIONS TO REGIONAL ANAESTHESIA

- Allergy to local anaesthetic
- Rejection of technique by patient
- Clinically manifest severe coagulation disorders
- Infection or haematoma at injection site
- Lack of experience with performing nerve block
- Relative contraindication: neurological defects (previous documentation necessary).

Systemic effects of local anaesthetic intoxication

See Figure 1.27.

Management of local anaesthetic toxicity

The Association of Anaesthetists of Great Britain and Ireland (AAGBI) Safety Guideline for Management of Severe Local Anaesthetic Toxicity is a guideline that outlines the steps for recognition, immediate management, and treatment of cases of local anaesthetic toxicity.[14]

Local anaesthetic toxicity may occur some time after the initial injection and may be recognized by several signs:[14]

- Alteration of mental status, severe agitation, or loss of consciousness:
  - May be associated with tonic-clonic convulsions
- Cardiovascular collapse:
  - Sinus bradycardia, conduction blocks, asystole, and ventricular tachyarrhythmias possible.

Treatment of local anaesthetic toxicity[14]

- Immediately, stop injection of local anaesthetic, and call for help
- Maintain the airway, securing with a tracheal tube, if necessary
- Give 100% oxygen, ensuring adequate lung ventilation
- Confirm/establish intravenous access
- Control seizures with a benzodiazepine, thiopental, or propofol, administered in small incremental doses
- Monitor cardiovascular status throughout
- If circulatory arrest occurs:
  - Start cardiopulmonary resuscitation (CPR), using standard protocols
  - Manage arrhythmias:
    - Arrhythmias may be very refractory to treatment
    - Do not use lignocaine
  - Administer intravenous lipid emulsion, according to protocol outlined under Treatment of local anaesthetic toxicity with intravenous lipid emulsion:

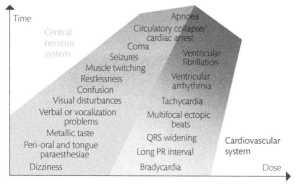

FIGURE 1.27 Symptoms and signs of local anaesthetic toxicity.

Adapted from Meier G & Büttner J. Regional anaesthesia. Pocket compendium of peripheral nerve blocks. 3rd edn. Munich: Acris Publishing Company, 2005.

- Continue CPR throughout administration
- Propofol is not a suitable substitute for lipid emulsion
- Recovery from cardiac arrest may take over 1 hour.
- If circulatory arrest does not occur:
  - Use conventional therapies to treat hypotension, bradycardia, and tachyarrhythmia
    - Do not use lignocaine.

Treatment of local anaesthetic toxicity with intravenous lipid emulsion[14]

Immediately:

- Inject an initial intravenous bolus of 20% lipid emulsion (1.5 mL/kg body weight) over 1 minute, and
- Start an intravenous infusion of 20% lipid emulsion (0.25 mL/kg body weight per minute, equivalent to 15 mL/kg body weight per hour).

After 5 minutes:

- A maximum of two repeat boluses of 20% lipid emulsion (1.5 mL/kg body weight) should be given if:
  - Cardiovascular stability has not been restored, or
  - Adequate circulation deteriorates
- Continue the infusion at the same rate, but double the rate to 0.50 mL/kg body weight per minute (30 mL/kg body weight per hour) at any time after 5 minutes, if:
  - Cardiovascular stability has not been restored, or
  - Adequate circulation deteriorates.

Other points to note:

- A maximum of three boluses may be given, including the initial bolus
- Leave 5 minutes between boluses
- Do not exceed a maximum cumulative dose of 12 mL/kg
- Following initial recovery, the patient should be transferred for appropriate further monitoring until sustained recovery is achieved
- Cases of local anaesthetic toxicity should be reported appropriately
- A quick reference guide to treatment of local anaesthetic toxicity is located on p.152.

Allergic reactions

Allergy for amide local anaesthetics is extremely rare and should be treated like any allergic reaction.

Post-operative analgesia

Injectable local anaesthetics

Concentrations, dosages, and durations of various injectable local anaesthetics
are given in Tables 1.1 and 1.2, and Figure 1.28. Box 1.3 details the special
features of some of these drugs.

Care of catheters for continuous infusions

- At least once a day:
  - Check the catheter position and insertion site for infection
  - Assess effectiveness of analgesia
  - Analyse indications critically
  - Document carefully.

- If analgesia is insufficient:
  - Check that the catheter is positioned correctly and has not dislodged
  - Inject bolus (e.g. 10 mL 0.2% ropivacaine) if analgesia is only partially
    effective
  - Provide supplementary analgesics (NSAID, paracetamol, opioids orally),
    as needed
  - Provide additional pain medication when removing the catheter.

- Duration of treatment:
  - Usually up to 3–5 days, depending on the indication (for chronic pain
    therapy, a duration of more than 100 days has been described)
  - An analgesic catheter can be used in outpatients, but the corresponding
    prerequisites must be considered.

TABLE 1.1 Concentration and recommended dosage[17–19]

	Bupivacaine	Lignocaine	Ropivacaine
Single injection			
Concentration	0.25–0.5%	1–2%	0.5–1%
Dosage*	Up to 2 mg/kg	Up to 4 mg/kg	Up to 2.5 mg/kg
Time until effective	10–25 min	5–15 min	10–25 min
Analgesic duration	Up to 12 h	2–5 h	Up to 12 h
Continuous infusion			
Concentration	0.125–0.25%	NA	0.2%
Dosage*	Up to 18.75 mg/h	NA	Up to 28 mg/h

NA, not administered for continuous infusions.
* The anaesthetist's experience and knowledge of the patient's physical status are important
determinants when calculating the anaesthetic dose to be administered.

TABLE 1.2 Pharmacokinetic profile following experimental intravenous administration in adults[17-19]

	Bupivacaine	Lignocaine	Ropivacaine
Total plasma clearance (L/min)	0.58	0.95	0.44
Steady-state distribution volume (L)	73	91	47
Elimination half-life in plasma (h)	2.7	1.6	1.8
Intermediate hepatic extraction ratio	0.40	0.65	0.40

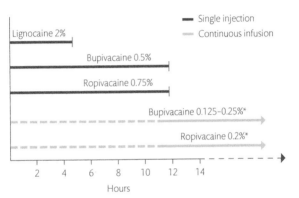

FIGURE 1.28 Analgesic duration of bupivacaine, lignocaine, and ropivacaine.
* Start infusion before the onset of post-operative pain; otherwise, start with an initial bolus.

BOX 1.3 SPECIAL FEATURES

Bupivacaine
- Long duration of action and slow onset.[15]

Lignocaine
- Produces a rapid onset of intense motor and sensory nerve blockade.[16]

Ropivacaine
- Long duration of action and slow onset[15]
- Reduced cardiovascular and CNS toxicity, compared with racemic bupivacaine.[16]

References

1 Australian and New Zealand College of Anaesthetists. Recommendations on the pre-anaesthesia consultation. Viewed 24 January 2010, <http://www.anzca.edu.au/resources/professional-documents/professional-standards/pdfs/PS7-2008.pdf>.

2 Oranje A and de Waard-van der Spek F (1995). Use of EMLA cream in dermatosurgical interventions of skin and genital mucosa. In: Koren G, ed. *Eutectic Mixture of Local Anesthetics (EMLA)*, pp. 123–36. New York: Marcel Dekker, Inc.

3 Tsui B and Kropelin B (2005). The electrophysiological effect of dextrose 5% in water on single-shot peripheral nerve stimulation. *Anesth Analg* **100**, 1837–9.

4 Australian and New Zealand College of Anaesthetists. Recommendations on monitoring during anaesthesia. Viewed 24 January 2010, <http://www.anzca.edu.au/resources/professional-documents/professional-standards/pdfs/PS18-2008.pdf>.

5 Marhofer P, Greher M, Kapral S (2005). Ultrasound guidance in regional anaesthesia. *Br J Anaesth* **94**, 7–17.

6 Gray A (2006). Ultrasound-guided regional anaesthesia. Current state of the art. *Anesthesiology* **104**, 368–73.

7 Chuan A (2007). Ultrasound guided regional anaesthesia. In: Ashley C, Chuan A, George L, Harrison J, eds. *Ultrasound in anaesthetic practice. Training manual.* 2nd edn, pp. 23–54. Sydney: Westmead Hospital Anaesthetic Department.

8 Neal J, Brull R, Chan V, *et al.* (2010). The ASRA evidence-based medicine assessment of ultrasound-guided regional anesthesia and pain medicine. Executive summary. *Reg Anesth Pain Med* **35**, S1–S9.

9 Perlas A and Chan V. Ultrasound-assisted nerve blocks. New York: New York School of Regional Anaesthesia. Viewed 19 October 2009, <http://www.nysora.com/peripheral_nerve_blocks/ultrasound-guided_techniques/3063-ultrasound_assisted_nerve_blocks.html>.

10 Hebbard P, Barrington M, Royse C. Ultrasound guided procedures in anaesthesia 2nd edn. Parkville: HeartWeb. Viewed 19 October 2009, <http://www.heartweb.com.au/>.

11 Australian and New Zealand College of Anaesthetists. Review Professional Standards 3—Guidelines for the management of major regional analgesia. Viewed 21 December 2009, <http://www.anzca.edu.au/resources/professional-documents/professional-standards/pdfs/PS3.pdf>.

12 Australasian Regional Anaesthesia Collaboration. 7-day follow up pathway. Viewed 20 October 2009, <http://www.regional.anaesthesia.org.au/>.

13 Horlocker T, Wedel D, Rowlingson J, *et al.* (2010). Regional anesthesia in the patient receiving antithrombotic or thrombolytic therapy: American Society of Regional Anesthesia and Pain Medicine evidence-based guidelines (3rd edn). *Reg Anesth Pain Med* **35**, 64–101.

14 Association of Anaesthetists of Great Britain & Ireland. AAGBI Safety guideline: Management of severe local anaesthetic toxicity. London: AAGBI. Viewed 1 February 2010, <http://www.aagbi.org/publications/guidelines/docs/la_toxicity_2010.pdf>.

15 Tetzlaff J (2000). The pharmacology of local anaesthetics. *Anesth Clin North America* **18**, 217–33.

16 McLure H and Rubin A (2005). Review of local anaesthetics. *Minerva Anestesiol* **71**, 59–74.

17 Naropin®. Australian Approved Product Information. 10 September 2010.

18 Xylocaine® Plain and Xylocaine® with Adrenaline. Australian Approved Product Information. 20 September 2010.

19 Marcain® and Marcain® with adrenaline. Australian Approved Product Information. 20 September 2010.

CHAPTER TWO
THE HEAD

Anatomy of the nerve supply to the head and scalp

The trigeminal ganglion (the fifth cranial nerve) is divided into sensory and motor branches. The ophthalmic and maxillary nerves are purely sensory. The mandibular nerve has both sensory and motor functions. These branches provide innervation to the face, scalp to the top of the head, conjunctiva, eye, paranasal sinuses, oral cavity, teeth, and dura. See Figure 2.1.

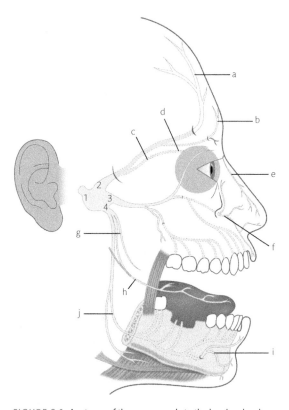

FIGURE 2.1 Anatomy of the nerve supply to the head and scalp.

1	Trigeminal n. ganglion	a	Supraorbital n.
2	Ophthalmic n.	b	Supratrochlear n.
3	Maxillary n.	c	Nasociliary n.
4	Mandibular n.	d	Anterior ethmoidal n.
		e	Anterior ethmoidal n. (external nasal branch)
		f	Infraorbital n.
		g	Buccal n.
		h	Lingual n.
		i	Mental n.
		j	Inferior alveolar n.

Sensory supply

See Figure 2.2.

FIGURE 2.2 Sensory
supply of the head
and scalp.

Divisions of the
trigeminal nerve:

V1 Ophthalmic area
V2 Maxillary area
V3 Mandibular area

Cervical plexus:

1   Greater occipital area
    (posterior division
    of C2)

2   Lesser occipital area
    (posterior division
    of C2)

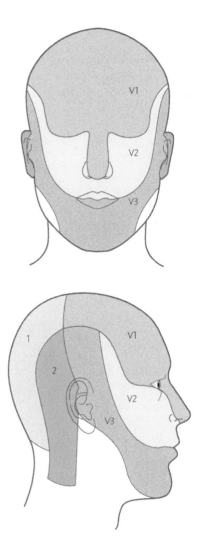

Peribulbar block

COMPLEXITY: ⬤⬤◯

Indications
- Anaesthesia and analgesia for eye surgery (e.g. cataract extraction, trabeculectomy, vitrectomy, and strabismus repair).

Specific contraindications
- Penetrating eye injury
- Scleromalacia
- Severe coagulopathy
- Axial length is >26 mm.

See Figures 2.3 to 2.5.

Technique
Patient position: supine. Ask the patient to look directly ahead and focus on a fixed point of the ceiling. This will ensure neutral positioning of the eyes.

Landmark: inferior orbital rim.

Technique: anaesthetize the conjunctiva by instilling three drops of 1% amethocaine or oxybuprocaine into the eye. Repeat three times at 1-minute intervals, if required. Clean the lower eyelid with half-strength iodine solution. At the lateral one-third and medial two-thirds junction of the inferior orbital rim, insert the needle percutaneously through the lower eyelid. Direct and advance the needle sagittally, parallel to the orbital floor and under the globe, until the needle hub is at the same depth as the iris (no more than 31 mm beyond the orbital rim). A distinctive 'pop' may be felt as the needle passes through the lower orbital septum. Following negative aspiration, inject 10–15 mL of anaesthetic solution slowly. Close the eye with adhesive tape, and apply gentle pressure for 5–10 minutes (manually or with an oculopressor) to lower intraocular pressure and allow spread of local anaesthetic.

Needle: 25 G, 2.5 cm.

Local anaesthetic: 0.75% or 1% ropivacaine with 75–150 U/mL hyaluronidase.

Comments: infiltration of the skin at the injection site with 0.5 mL 1% lignocaine improves patient comfort. Advantages of peribulbar anaesthesia over retrobulbar anaesthesia include reduced incidence of retrobulbar haemorrhage, optic nerve and globe damage, and intradural injection. A single injection is usually sufficient for anaesthesia and is easy to perform. If insufficient, a second superior injection is required.[1] Hyaluronidase is commonly added to facilitate anaesthetic spread. Less than 10 mL of ropivacaine is required for anaesthesia if 300 U/mL of hyaluronidase is added. A total of 8 mL of a 1:1 mixture of 2.0% lignocaine and 0.5% bupivacaine (with 75–150 U/mL hyaluronidase) can also be injected.[2] Potential disadvantages of combining anaesthetic agents include bacterial contamination, substitution errors, and limited shelf life.

FIGURE 2.3 Muscles in the region of the eye.

1 Medial rectus m.
2 Superior rectus m.
3 Superior oblique m.
4 Needle insertion site
5 Inferior oblique m.
6 Lateral rectus m.
7 Inferior rectus m.

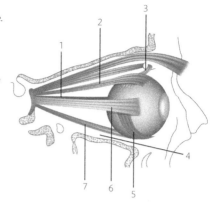

FIGURE 2.4 Insert the needle at the lateral one-third and medial two-thirds junction of the inferior orbital rim.

a Needle insertion site

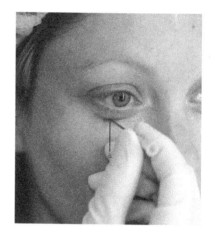

FIGURE 2.5 Direct and advance the needle sagitally, parallel to the orbital floor and under the globe.

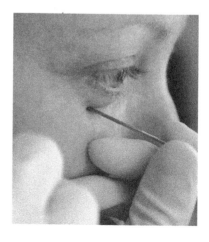

Sub-Tenon's eye block

COMPLEXITY: ⬤⬤⬤

Tenon's capsule is a layer of elastic white connective tissue that surrounds the globe deep to the conjunctiva. Anteriorly, it merges with the conjunctiva, approximately 1 mm from the limbus, and extends posteriorly to attach to a fibrous ring around the optic nerve. A potential space between the Tenon's capsule and the sclera is the sub-Tenon space.

Indications

- Anaesthesia and analgesia for eye surgery (e.g. cataract extraction, trabeculectomy, vitrectomy, and strabismus repair).

Specific contraindications

- Penetrating eye injury
- Scleromalacia.

See Figures 2.6 to 2.8.

Technique

Patient position: supine. To expose the inferonasal quadrant of the anterior eye, ask the patient to look up and out over their ipsilateral shoulder.

Landmarks: inferonasal quadrant and limbus.

Technique: anaesthetize the conjunctiva by instilling three drops of 1% amethocaine or oxybuprocaine into the eye. Prepare the eye with half-strength povidone-iodine solution. Place a wire lid speculum to hold the eyelids open. Using Moorefields forceps, lift the conjunctiva (and underlying Tenon's capsule) in the inferonasal quadrant, and make a small incision with Wescott spring scissors through the conjunctiva approximately 5 mm from the limbus. White bare sclera should be visible through the cut. While lifting the conjunctiva, gently advance the closed scissors through the incision to blunt dissect anterior adhesions between the Tenon's capsule and the sclera. Remove scissors, and insert the sub-Tenon cannula (with syringe attached) through the incision, and gently advance, following the curvature of the globe. Beyond the equator of the globe, clear adhesions that may hinder the passage of the cannula by gentle hydrodissection. Infuse 5 mL of anaesthetic slowly when the cannula is fully inserted. Close the eyelid on removing the cannula, and apply gentle direct digital pressure to the insertion point (or oculopressure device 35 mmHg for 5 minutes). The anaesthetic will initially fill the sub-Tenon's space, then pass posteriorly into the retrobulbar space and eventually into the extraconal space. Complete akinesia and anaesthesia should occur within 5 minutes. Ptosis commonly occurs with injection of 5 mL of anaesthetic.

Needle: 19 G, 25 mm sub-Tenon cannula (blunt, flattened, and curved).

Local anaesthetic: 2% lignocaine, 0.5% bupivacaine, or 0.75–1% ropivacaine with 60–300 U/mL hyaluronidase.

Comments: as this block requires a low volume of anaesthetic and minimal pressure, surgery can proceed rapidly as changes in intraocular pressure are minimal.[3] The addition of hyaluronidase facilitates the speed of onset of anaesthesia.[4] This block is more comfortable than peribulbar block and as effective as retrobulbar block, without the risks of retrobulbar haemorrhage, nerve or globe injury, or subdural injection.[5]

FIGURE 2.6 Anatomy
for sub-Tenon's eye block

1   Levator palpebral
    superioris m.
2   Superior rectus m.
3   Connective tissue
    bands
4   Optic n.
5   Bulbar fascia
6   Inferior rectus m.
7   Cornea
8   Superior tarsus
9   Lens
10 Inferior tarsus

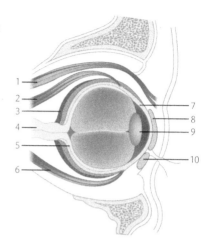

FIGURE 2.7 Insert
the sub-Tenon cannula
through the inferonasal
incision.

a   Needle insertion site

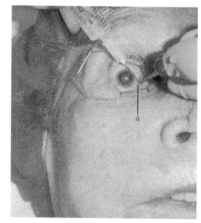

FIGURE 2.8 The
sub-Tenon cannula is
fully inserted.

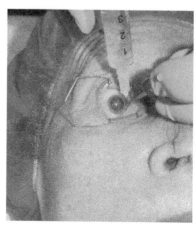

Supraorbital and supratrochlear nerve block

COMPLEXITY: ✪✪✪

Indications
- Anaesthesia and analgesia for lower forehead and upper eyelid surgery (e.g. excision of skin lesions, suturing of lacerations).

Side effects and complications
- Periorbital ecchymosis (black eye; uncommon).[6]

See Figures 2.9 and 2.10.

Technique
Patient position: supine.

Landmark: supraorbital ridge.

Technique: insert the needle in the midline just above the supraorbital ridge, and raise a bleb of local anaesthetic. Inject 3–4 mL of anaesthetic subcutaneously and slowly along the supraorbital ridge in a lateral direction to block both the supraorbital and supratrochlear nerves. Repeat on the opposing side to block the nerve bilaterally.

Needle: 25 G, 38 mm.

Local anaesthetic: 2% lignocaine with adrenaline 1:200 000, 0.5% bupivacaine or 0.75–1% ropivacaine.

Comments: lignocaine with adrenaline provides surgical anaesthesia for up to 3 hours and analgesia for 6–9 hours. Prior to injecting lignocaine with adrenaline, cover the patient's eye with an eye pad to prevent adrenaline from seeping onto the eye.[6] As injections in the face can cause anxiety in patients, it is important to be gentle, inject anaesthetic slowly and carefully, and wait for a result. An anxiolytic, such as midazolam, may be given to patients to reduce their anxiety.

FIGURE 2.9 The supraorbital, infraorbital, and mental foramen align parasagittally on the face.

a   Needle insertion site

b   Inject the local anaesthetic to midpoint of supraorbital ridge

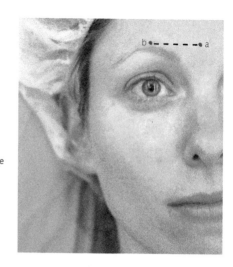

FIGURE 2.10

1   Supraorbital n.

2   Supratrochlear n.

3   Supraorbital foramen

4   Orbital cavity

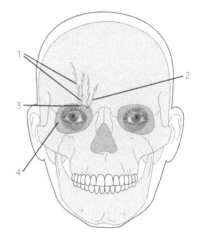

Infraorbital nerve block

Indications

- Anaesthesia and analgesia for upper lip, lower eyelid and cheek surgery (e.g. excision of skin lesions and suturing of lacerations).

Side effects and complications

- Minor bruising[6]
- Retrograde passage of the anaesthetic if injected into (rather than adjacent to) the infraorbital foramen, resulting in more generalized anaesthetic effects than expected.[6]

See Figures 2.11 to 2.13.

Technique

Patient position: supine.

Landmarks: extra-oral: infraorbital foramen; intra-oral: junction of alveolar and buccal mucosa.

Technique: for extra-oral injection, palpate the infraorbital foramen (1 cm below the midpoint of the inferior orbital margin). Insert the needle adjacent to the infraorbital foramen, and inject the anaesthetic slowly. For intra-oral injection, retract the upper lip with the thumb and forefinger. Insert the needle parallel to the face at the junction of the alveolar and buccal mucosa. Advance the needle gently through the mucosa for approximately 1 cm. Inject 1–2 mL of anaesthetic slowly.

Needle: 25 or 27 G, 10 mm.

Local anaesthetic: 2% lignocaine with adrenaline 1:200 000.

Comments: lignocaine with adrenaline provides surgical anaesthesia for up to 3 hours and analgesia for 6–9 hours. Injection of bupivacaine or ropivacaine is not recommended, as this will result in a lip that is heavily blocked for many hours. Direct infiltration of the operative site with lignocaine with adrenaline is a better alternative. As injections in the face can cause anxiety in patients, it is important to be gentle, inject slowly and carefully, and wait for a result. An anxiolytic, such as midazolam, may be given to patients to reduce their anxiety. Warn patients to avoid hot drinks until the block has worn off.

FIGURE 2.11

1   Infraorbital foramen
2   Infraorbital n.

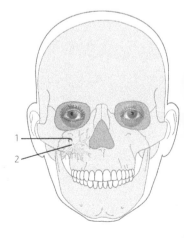

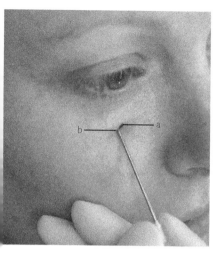

FIGURE 2.12 Extra-oral route: insert the needle adjacent to, but not into, the infraorbital foramen.

a   Infraorbital foramen   b   Needle insertion site

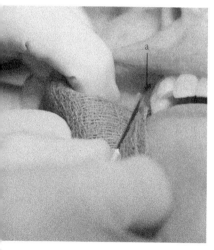

FIGURE 2.13 Intra-oral route: insert the needle into the gum at the junction of the alveolar and buccal mucosa.

a   Needle insertion site

Mental nerve block

COMPLEXITY: ★★★

Indications
- Anaesthesia and analgesia for the bottom lip and chin surgery (e.g. complete vermilionectomy, wedge resection).

Side effects and complications
- Minor bruising[6]
- Salivary drooling while the block is effective.[6]

See Figures 2.14 and 2.15.

Technique

Patient position: supine.

Landmark: mental foramen (located below the second premolar or between the first and second premolar teeth).

Technique: for intra-oral injection, insert the needle at the junction of the alveolar and buccal mucosa (topical lignocaine may be applied prior to injecting the anaesthetic). Advance the needle about 1 cm through the mucosa until it is over the mental foramen. Inject 1–2 mL of anaesthetic slowly. To perform full surgery of the lower lip, both inside and out, block the nerve bilaterally.

Needle: 25 G, 38 mm.

Local anaesthetic: 2% lignocaine with adrenaline 1:200 000.

Comments: lignocaine with adrenaline provides surgical anaesthesia for up to 3 hours and analgesia for 6–9 hours. As for infraorbital block, avoid injecting bupivacaine or ropivacaine, and infiltrate the operative site with lignocaine with adrenaline. Blocking the mental nerve does not anaesthetize the gums or teeth. As injections in the face can cause anxiety in patients, it is important to be gentle, inject slowly and carefully, and wait for a result. An anxiolytic, such as midazolam, may be given to patients to reduce their anxiety. Warn patients to avoid hot drinks until the block has worn off.

FIGURE 2.14

1   Mental foramen

2   Mental n.

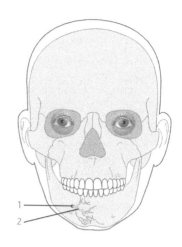

FIGURE 2.15

Insert the needle into the gum at the junction of the alveolar and buccal mucosa.

a   Needle insertion site

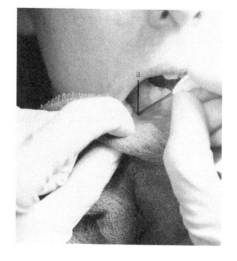

Maxillary nerve block

COMPLEXITY: ✪✪✪

Indications

- Anaesthesia and analgesia for maxillary teeth, buccal and palatal soft tissue as far as the midline, upper lip, lateral aspect of the nose, and the lower eyelid sugery (for nasal surgery, see Anterior ethmoidal nerve block)
- Supplemental anaesthesia for transphenoidal hypophysectomy.

Side effects and complications

- Haematoma formation.

See Figures 2.16 to 2.18.

Technique (lateral extra-oral approach)

Patient position: supine with head in neutral position.

Landmark: zygomatic arch (posterior and anterior limits) and lateral pterygoid plate.   .

Technique: palpate the zygomatic arch, and locate its posterior and anterior limits. To identify the posterior limit, ask the patient to open their mouth to feel the movement of the mandible head just in front of the tragus. The point at which the arch joins the posterior convexity of the zygomatic process of the maxilla is the anterior limit. Locate the midpoint on the inferior border of the arch by bisecting the length of the arch. Infiltrate the area with 2% lignocaine (2 mL). Insert and advance the needle (approximately 4–5 cm) until it contacts the lateral pterygoid plate. Note needle depth; place a 0.25 cm marker on the needle, and withdraw. Redirect the needle anteriorly and superiorly to pass anterior to the lateral pterygoid plate into the pterygopalatine fossa. Advance the needle no further than 0.25 cm deeper than the lateral pterygoid plate. Following negative aspiration, inject 5 mL of anaesthetic slowly.

Needle: 25 G, 10 cm, short bevel, or 22 G spinal needle.

Local anaesthetic: 2% lignocaine with adrenaline 1:200 000, or 0.75% ropivacaine.

FIGURE 2.16

1 Trigeminal ganglion
2 Maxillary n.
3 Pterygopalatine fossa
4 Zygomatic arch
5 Mandible

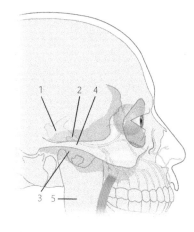

FIGURE 2.17 Insert and advance the needle until it contacts the lateral pterygoid plate.

a Midpoint of the inferior border of the zygomatic arch and needle insertion site

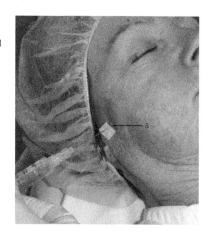

FIGURE 2.18 Redirect the needle anteriorly and superiorly to pass anterior to the lateral pterygoid plate into the pterygopalatine fossa.

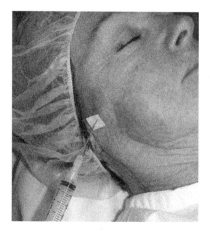

Anterior ethmoidal nerve block

COMPLEXITY: ✪✪✪

The anterior ethmoidal nerve is the terminal branch of the nasociliary nerve. It exits the skull into the orbit, re-enters through the anterior ethmoidal foramen, and runs along the cribriform plate and anteriorly down the nose.

Indications

• Anaesthesia and analgesia of the anterior third of the nose and nasal septum (use in conjunction with maxillary nerve block for nasal surgery).

Side effects and complications

• Periorbital haematoma.

See Figures 2.19 to 2.21.

Single injection technique

Patient position: supine with head in neutral position.

Landmark: orbital margin and inner canthus.

Technique: insert needle 1.5–2 cm lateral to the orbital margin and 1 cm above the inner canthus. Advance the needle 2 cm until it touches the medial orbital wall near the anterior ethmoidal foramen. Inject 3 mL of anaesthetic. Perform the block bilaterally.

Needle: 25 G, 2.5 cm.

Local anaesthetic: 2% lignocaine with adrenaline 1:200 000, or 0.75% ropivacaine.

FIGURE 2.19

1 Nasociliary n.
2 Anterior ethmoidal n.
3 Anterior ethmoidal foramen
4 Infratrochear n. (from
   nasociliary n.)
5 Anterior ethmoidal
   n. (external nasal branch)

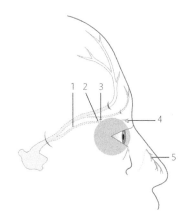

FIGURE 2.20

a Anterior ethmoidal
   foramen

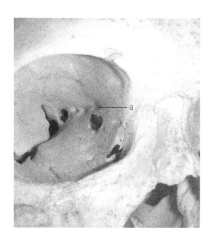

FIGURE 2.21

Insert the needle lateral
to the orbital margin
and above the inner
canthus.

a Needle insertion site

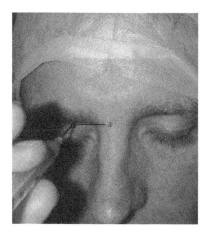

References

1 Hendrick S, Rosenberg M, Lebenbom-Mansour M (1997). Efficacy and safety of single injection peribulbar block performed by anesthesiologists prior to cataract surgery. *J Clin Anesth* **9**, 285–8.

2 Corke P, Baker J, Cammack R (1999). Comparison of 1% ropivacaine and a mixture of 2% lignocaine and 0.5% bupivacaine for peribulbar anaesthesia in cataract surgery. *Anaesth Intensive Care* **27**, 249–52.

3 Verma S and Makker R (2001). Sub-Tenon eye block: approaching the ideal? [letter]. *Anesthesiology* **94**, 376–7.

4 Guise P and Laurent S (1999). Sub-Tenon's block: the effect of hyaluronidase on speed of onset and block quality. *Anaesth Intensive Care* **27**, 179–81.

5 Davison M, Padroni S, Bunce C, Rüschen H (2007). Sub-Tenon's anaesthesia versus topical anaesthesia for cataract surgery (review). *Cochrane Database Syst Rev* **3**, CD006291.

6 Simpson S (2001). Regional nerve blocks. Part 2—the face and scalp. *Aust Fam Physician* **30**, 565–8.

CHAPTER THREE

UPPER EXTREMITIES

Anatomy of the brachial plexus

The brachial plexus is formed by the anterior primary rami of the C5 to T1 (variably C4 and T2) spinal nerves and runs from the vertebral column between the clavicle and the first rib. The brachial plexus enters the upper limb in the axilla before dividing into four main terminal branches: the median, radial, ulnar, and musculocutaneous nerves. See Figure 3.1.

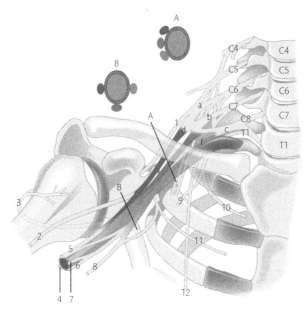

FIGURE 3.1 Anatomy of the brachial plexus. Inset A and B: sectional plane in the infraclavicular and axillary region. Note the position of the cords.

a	Superior trunk (rami ventrales C5 and C6)	3	Axillary n.
		4	Radial n.
b	Middle trunk (ramus ventralis C7)	5	Median n.
c	Inferior trunk (rami ventrales C8 and T1)	6	Ulnar n.
		7	Medial antebrachial cutaneous n.
d	Lateral cord	8	Medial brachial cutaneous n.
e	Posterior cord	9	Intercostobrachial n.
f	Medial cord	10	Intercostal n. I
		11	Intercostal n. II
1	Suprascapular n.	12	Long thoracic n.
2	Musculocutaneous n.		

Sensory supply

See Figure 3.2.

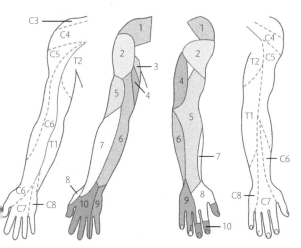

FIGURE 3.2 Sensory supply of the arm and hand.

1 Supraclavicular n.
2 Axillary n. (lateral cutaneous brachial n.)
3 Intercostobrachial n.
4 Medial brachial cutaneous n.
5 Posterior antebrachial cutaneous n. (radial n.)
6 Medial antebrachial cutaneous n.
7 Lateral antebrachial cutaneous n. (musculocutaneous n.)
8 Radial n.
9 Ulnar n.
10 Median n.

Motor response

See Figure 3.3.

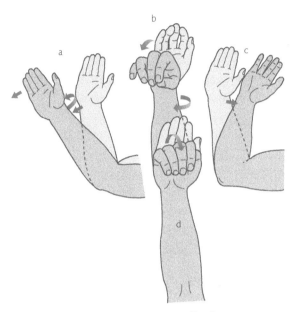

FIGURE 3.3 Motor response of the arm and hand.

a   Radial n.: stretching elbow and fingers
b   Median n.: flexion of the fingers
c   Musculocutaneous n.: flexion (and supination) of the forearm
d   Ulnar n.: flexion of the fourth and fifth fingers, with opposition of the first finger

Scanning tips for the upper extremities

Brachial plexus

Imaging of the brachial plexus is best achieved with high-frequency linear probes with a range of 10–15 MHz, although probes with a range of 4–7 MHz may be required for the infraclavicular region where the plexus cords may be more deeply located.[1]

Interscalene

The cervical nerve roots that form the brachial plexus are located between the anterior and middle scalene muscles. Scanning the lateral aspect of the neck in an axial oblique plane is the best approach for visualizing these nerve roots. Identify the sternocleidomastoid muscle superficially, and the anterior and middle scalene muscles deeper. In the interscalene groove, visualize one or more nerve roots as mostly hypoechoic structures with some internal punctuate echoes. The vertebral artery and vein are seen alongside the transverse spinous processes deeper again, while the carotid artery and internal jugular veins are located medially and anteriorly.[1] See Figure 3.4.

Supraclavicular/infraclavicular

Use a linear probe in a coronal oblique plane to scan the brachial plexus in the supraclavicular region. Identify the subclavian artery immediately superior to the first rib; the anterior and middle scalene muscles as they insert on the first rib; and the pleura immediately deep to the first rib. Posterior and cephalad to the subclavian artery, the divisions of the brachial plexus are visualized tightly arranged and may have the appearance of a bunch of dark grapes. The plexus may be somewhat spread out, with the C7 trunk between the first rib and the artery.[1]

If the anatomy is unclear, the plexus may be confirmed by scanning in a caudad-cephalad motion, following the hypoechoic roots and trunks along their paths.

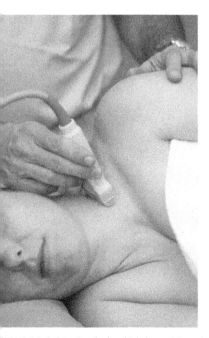

FIGURE 3.4 Scanning the brachial plexus—interscalene.

For the infraclavicular approach, use a linear probe with a range of 4–7 MHz in a parasagittal plane immediately medial to the coracoid process. The cords of the plexus lie deep to the pectoralis major and pectoralis minor muscles and appear hyperechoic in a transverse view adjacent to the axillary vessels. For orientation in larger patients, it may be helpful to commence scanning at the midpoint of the clavicle. The plexus here is generally located cephaloposterior to the artery; the lateral cord is cephalad to the artery, while the posterior cord is posterior to the artery. The medial cord is often—but not always—identified between the artery and vein.[1]

See Figures 3.5 and 3.6.

Axillary

The terminal branches of the brachial plexus, including the musculocutaneous, median, ulnar, and radial nerves, are located superficially in the axilla and the upper arm within the bicipital sulcus.[1]

Abduct the arm 90°, and flex the forearm. Use a linear 10-15 MHz probe, positioned as close to the axilla as possible, perpendicular to the long axis of the arm. Identify the round pulsatile axillary artery in the bicipital sulcus, distinguishable from the axillary veins that are readily compressed. Visualize the round to oval-shaped hypoechoic nerves in the axilla, with the hyperechoic epineurium within. In this region, the median nerve is usually medial to the artery, while the ulnar nerve is lateral. The location of the radial nerve is highly variable but is often posterior or posterolateral to the artery. More proximally, the musculocutaneous nerve branches off and may be visualized as a hyperechoic structure between the biceps and coracobrachialis muscles before it enters the body of the coracobrachialis muscle.[1]

Local anaesthetic should be injected individually around each nerve for most consistent results when performing an axillary block. It is presumed that the spread of local anaesthetic within the sheath compartment is restricted by the septae.[1]

See Figure 3.7.

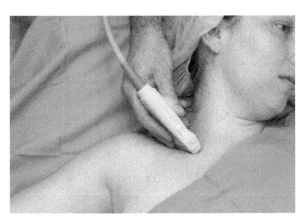

FIGURE 3.5 Scanning the brachial plexus—supraclavicular.

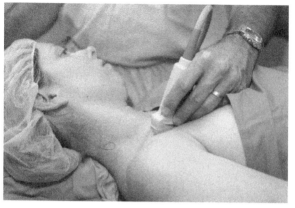

FIGURE 3.6 Scanning the brachial plexus—infraclavicular.

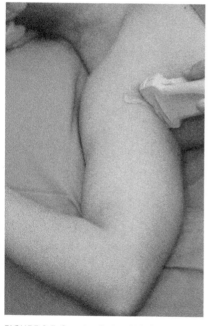

FIGURE 3.7 Scanning the brachial plexus—axillary.

Interscalene plexus block

COMPLEXITY: ⬤⬤⬤

Indications
- Anaesthesia and analgesia for open and arthroscopic shoulder surgery (e.g. acromioplasties, total shoulder replacements, debridement of labral and rotator cuff tears)
- Mobilization (e.g. frozen shoulder)
- Physiotherapy in the shoulder region
- Therapy for pain syndromes
- Sympathicolysis.

Specific contraindications
- Contralateral phrenic and recurrent paresis
- Chronic obstructive pulmonary disease (relative contraindication).

Side effects and complications
- Spread of anaesthetic to other tissues that may manifest as ipsilateral numbness of the face, recurrent laryngeal nerve block resulting in variable paralysis of the vocal cord,[2] Horner's syndrome (unequal pupils; 100%),[2] or variable ipsilateral phrenic nerve block[3]
- Vertebral artery injection
- Subarachnoid injection
- Epidural injection
- Pneumothorax.

See Figures 3.8, 3.9 and 3.10.

Single injection technique[4]
Patient position: supine, with head rotated away from the side to be blocked. Place the ipsilateral arm on the patient's lap. It may be helpful to sit patients with a short neck upright. In thin patients, the plexus may be palpated as a ropy structure running medial to lateral towards the shoulder.

Landmarks: sternocleidomastoid muscle (lateral border), scalenus anterior muscle, interscalene groove, and cricoid cartilage.

Technique: with the patient's head elevated slightly, palpate the lateral border of the sternocleidomastoid muscle, and place the index and middle fingers of the non-injecting hand immediately behind this muscle. Ask the patient to relax so that the palpating fingers move medially behind this muscle and come to rest on the belly of the scalenus anterior muscle. Roll fingers laterally across this muscle until the interscalene groove is palpated. In many patients, the plexus may be palpated as a firm band running from medial to lateral in the neck. Insert the needle in the interscalene groove, 2 cm cephalad to the cricoid cartilage. Direct the needle caudad and laterally (towards the middle third of the contralateral clavicle) along the interscalene groove at a 30° angle to the skin. Twitching of the deltoid and/or biceps brachii muscles at a stimulating current of 0.3 mA/0.1 ms indicates correct needle placement. Inject 20–30 mL of anaesthetic slowly (initial injection may be uncomfortable).

Needle: 22 G, 2–4 cm, short bevel, insulated.

Local anaesthetic: 1% lignocaine (30 mL), 0.5% bupivacaine, or 0.75% ropivacaine.

Comments: Meier's approach differs to the classical interscalene plexus block described by Winnie (1970) in that the needle is inserted 1–2 cm cephalad from that described by Winnie, and is directed.

FIGURE 3.8

a Sternocleidomastoid m.
b Interscalene groove
c Subclavian a.

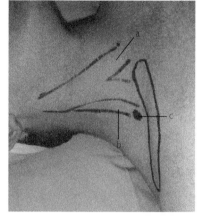

FIGURE 3.9

1 Sternocleidomastoid m.
2 Phrenic n.
3 Scalenus medius m.
4 Brachial plexus (supraclavicular)
5 Scalenus anterior m.
6 Omohyoid m.
7 Brachial plexus (infraclavicular)
8 Subclavian a.
9 External jugular v.
10 Internal jugular v.
11 Cricoid cartilage

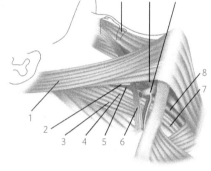

FIGURE 3.10 Insert the needle in the interscalene groove.

a Needle insertion site

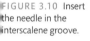

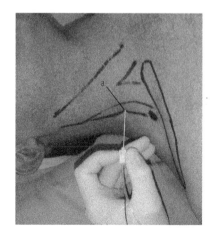

Interscalene plexus block

Laterally, rather than medially, dorsally and caudad, and approaches the brachial plexus at a more tangential angle, rather than at a right angle. As the plexus is superficial (usually no deeper than 2 cm), most complications are caused by advancing the needle tip too deeply. Contraction of the levator scapulae muscle with stimulation indicates the needle has been directed too posteriorly, whereas contraction of the diaphragm (phrenic nerve) indicates the needle has been directed too anteriorly.

See Figures 3.11, 3.12, and 3.13.

Continuous catheter technique

Technique: locate the interscalene groove, as described for the single injection technique. Insert the needle in a more cephalad position and direct caudad. Perform the continuous catheter technique, as described under Catheter technique for continuous infusions.

Equipment: StimuCath™, or Plexolong or Contiplex® (19.5 G, 3–6 cm, insulated Tuohy needle and wire-stiffened 20 G catheter).

Local anaesthetic: 0.2% ropivacaine.

Ultrasound-guided technique

Patient position: lateral, with side to be blocked uppermost.

Landmarks: surface: larynx and sternocleidomastoid muscle; sonoanatomical: thyroid gland, carotid artery, and internal jugular vein.

Technique: place the ultrasound probe lateral to the larynx, and visualize the thyroid gland, the carotid artery, and the internal jugular vein. Move the probe sideways to the lateral border of the sternocleidomastoid muscle while moving the tip of the probe slightly caudad. In the SAX view, the brachial plexus will become visible as multiple round or oval hypoechoic areas between the scalenus anterior and scalenus medius muscles. Using an IP approach, insert the needle from posterior, advancing through the scalenus medius muscle into the interscalene groove. Confirm needle placement with a test dose of anaesthetic, then inject 10–15 mL (maximum 20 mL) of anaesthetic, observing spread around nerve roots. If placing a catheter, pass it 1–2 cm beyond the needle tip under vision, and withdraw needle. Dose through catheter, observing local anaesthetic spread; small volumes may be required.

Needle: 22 G, 4 cm with a facette tip.

Local anaesthetic: 1% lignocaine, 0.5% bupivacaine, 0.75% ropivacaine, or 1:1 mixture of 2% lignocaine and 1% ropivacaine.

Comments: in some patients, a scalenus intermedius muscle or fascial layer may divide the plexus into a more superficial (upper trunk) and deeper (middle and lower trunks) structure. Phrenic nerve block is minimized, as the spread of local anaesthetic out of the interscalene groove can be avoided. To block the entire brachial plexus, slightly reposition the needle to include the T1 root.[5] The T1 root forms part of the ulnar nerve and is not blocked by nerve stimulation guidance.

FIGURE 3.11 Insert the
needle from posterior,
using an IP approach.

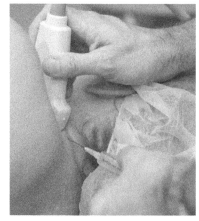

FIGURE 3.12 SAX view
of the interscalene.

a   Sternocleidomastoid

b   Interscalene plexus

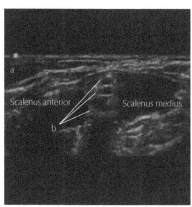

FIGURE 3.13 SAX view
of the interscalene.

a   Sternocleidomastoid

b   Interscalene plexus

c   Carotid a.

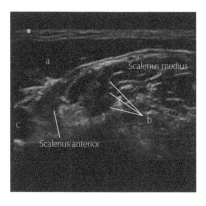

Supraclavicular plexus block

COMPLEXITY: ✪✪✪

Indications
• Anaesthesia and analgesia for upper and lower arm, and hand surgery.

Specific contraindications
• Severe chronic airways disease (relative).

Side effects and complications
• Pneumothorax
• Phrenic nerve block
• Horner's syndrome
• Subclavian artery puncture
• Haemothorax.

See Figures 3.14, 3.15, and 3.16.

Single injection technique

Patient position: semi-sitting, with the head elevated and rotated 30° away from the arm to be blocked.

Landmarks: interscalene groove and subclavian artery.

Technique: palpate the lateral border of the sternocleidomastoid muscle, and place the index and middle fingers of the non-injecting hand immediately behind this muscle. Ask the patient to relax so that the palpating fingers move medially behind this muscle and come to rest on the belly of the scalenus anterior muscle. Roll fingers laterally across this muscle until the interscalene groove is palpated. Palpate the interscalene groove caudad until the subclavian artery is felt above the clavicle (50% of patients). Place a finger on the artery, and insert a needle into the posterior part of the groove and posterior to the subclavian artery. With the needle hub against the neck, direct the needle caudad and parallel to the midline. Advance the needle to the plexus. Stimulation will elicit flexion or extension of the fingers with correct needle placement. Inject 30–40 mL of anaesthetic slowly.

Needle: 22 G, 5 cm, short bevel, insulated.

Local anaesthetic: 1.5–2% lignocaine, 0.5% bupivacaine, or 0.75–1% ropivacaine.

Comments: unless contraindicated, a nerve stimulator-guided infraclavicular plexus block is the preferred approach. The supraclavicular plexus block has been included as a nerve stimulator-guided approach for completeness. The authors do not recommend this block without ultrasound guidance for inexperienced anaesthetists, as the risk of serious complications is relatively high. The patient's weight will influence the amount of pressure the palpating finger needs to exert. Palpation helps to reduce the distance between the brachial plexus and skin and decreases the needle trajectory. This technique should be avoided if the subclavian artery cannot be palpated. Continuous catheter technique is not recommended, as there is a risk of catheter dislodgement.

FIGURE 3.14

a Sternocleidomastoid m.
b Interscalene groove
c Subclavian a.

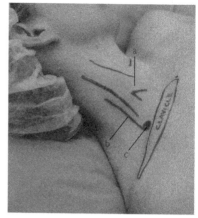

FIGURE 3.15

1 Sternocleidomastoid m.
2 Phrenic n.
3 Scalenus medius m.
4 Brachial plexus (supraclavicular)
5 Scalenus anterior m.
6 Omohyoid m.
7 Brachial plexus (infraclavicular)
8 Subclavian a.
9 External jugular v.
10 Internal jugular v.
11 Cricoid cartilage

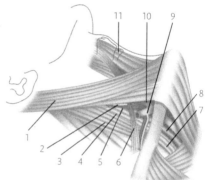

FIGURE 3.16 Direct the needle caudad and parallel to the midline, and advance to the plexus.

a Needle insertion site

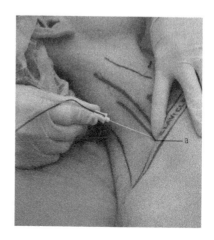

Supraclavicular plexus block

COMPLEXITY: ⚫⚫⚫
See Figures 3.17, 3.18, and 3.19.

Ultrasound-guided technique

Patient position: semi-sitting, with head rotated away from the arm to be blocked. The patient lowers their shoulder and flexes their elbow so that their forearm rests on their lap.

Landmarks: surface: supraclavicular fossa; sonoanatomical: subclavian artery and scalenus medius and scalenus anterior muscles.

Technique: place the ultrasound probe in the supraclavicular fossa (the posterior triangle of the neck bordered by the collarbone, the posterior margin of the sternocleidomastoid muscle, and the trapezius muscle) in an almost parasagittal plane. In most patients, the brachial plexus is cephaloposterior to the subclavian artery and may be seen between the scalenus medius and scalenus anterior muscles. Insert the needle, using either an IP or OOP approach. Initially, place the needle close to the first rib, and place initial dose to block the lower trunk, then reposition to block more superior trunks. Confirm needle placement with a test dose of anaesthetic, then inject up to 20 mL of anaesthetic slowly.

Needle: 22 or 24 G, 2.5–5 cm, short bevel.

Local anaesthetic: 1.5–2% lignocaine, 0.75–1% ropivacaine, or a 1:1 mixture of 2% lignocaine and 1% ropivacaine.

Comments: variation in the location of the brachial plexus at the supraclavicular level can be accommodated for by ultrasound, ensuring that all nerves that form the plexus are anaesthetized. In particular, carefully examine the region between the subclavian artery and the first rib for nerves, which may account for patchy blocks. Division of the plexus by vascular structures is also common, and, in the supraclavicular region, the dorsal scapular artery may divide the plexus. Ultrasound enables positioning of the planned needle trajectory away from vascular structures.

FIGURE 3.17 Insert the needle, using an (a) OOP approach or (b) IP approach.

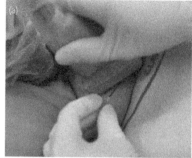

FIGURE 3.18 SAX view of the supraclavicular.

a   Subclavian a.
b   Pleura
c   Plexus
d   First rib

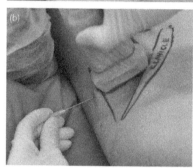

FIGURE 3.19 SAX view of the supraclavicular CFD.

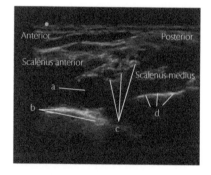

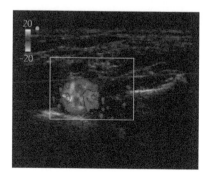

Infraclavicular plexus block: vertical approach

COMPLEXITY: ⭐⭐☆

Indications
- Anaesthesia and analgesia for upper arm, lower arm, and hand surgery
- Analgesia for physiotherapeutic treatment
- Treatment of pain syndrome
- Sympathicolysis.

Specific contraindications
- Thorax deformity
- Foreign bodies in the needle insertion area (e.g. pacemaker)
- Clavicular malunion.

Side effects and complications
- Intravascular injection
- Pneumothorax
- Horner's syndrome.

See Figures 3.20, 3.21, and 3.22.

Single injection technique

Patient position: supine.

Landmarks: acromion (ventral process) and clavicle.

Technique: palpate the ventral process of the acromion. Make a mark 2 cm caudad and 2 cm medial to this point. Direct the needle sagittally, and advance approximately 3 cm (or to the same depth as the middle of the head of the humerus, depending on patient habitus). Correct placement of the needle will elicit flexion of the fingers (median nerve) at a stimulating current of 0.3 mA/0.1 ms. Inject 30 mL of anaesthetic slowly.

Needle: 22 G, 4–6 cm, short bevel.

Local anaesthetic: 1.5% lignocaine (30–40 mL), 0.5% bupivacaine, or 0.75% ropivacaine.

Comments: risk of pneumothorax. To avoid, do not insert the needle too far medially or deviate from the sagittal direction of insertion. Always perform this block using a nerve stimulator. If stimulation induces twitching of the biceps brachii muscle only, withdraw needle to a subcutaneous position; shift it slightly lateral, and re-advance it in a strictly sagittal direction. As the musculocutaneous nerve exits the brachial sheath before the coracoid process, twitching only of the biceps brachii muscle indicates incorrect needle placement and yields poor results. Stimulation of the median nerve yields the best results.

Continuous catheter technique

Technique: locate the nerve as described above. Perform continuous catheter technique as described under Catheter technique for continuous infusions.

Equipment: StimuCath™, or Plexolong or Contiplex® (19.5 G, 3–6 cm, insulated Tuohy needle, and wire-stiffened 20 G catheter).

Local anaesthetic: 0.2% ropivacaine.

FIGURE 3.20

a Acromion (ventral
   process)
b Clavicle
c Needle insertion site

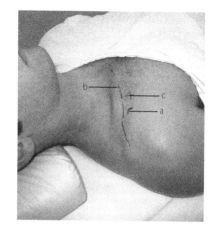

FIGURE 3.21

1 Pectoralis major m.
2 Subclavian a.
3 Pectoral n.
4 Brachial plexus
   (infraclavicular)
5 Deltoid m.
6 Suprascapular n.

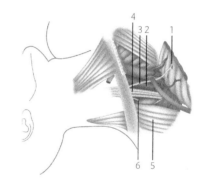

FIGURE 3.22 Direct
and advance the
needle approximately
3 cm sagitally.

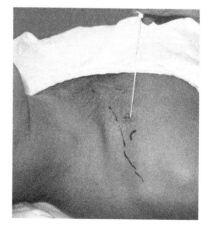

Infraclavicular plexus block: vertical approach

COMPLEXITY: ⚫⚫⚫
See Figures 3.23, 3.24, 3.25, and 3.26.

Ultrasound-guided technique

Patient position: supine, with arm by side. To position the brachial plexus more superficially, abduct the patient's arm over their head.

Landmarks: surface: deltopectoral triangle; sonoanatomical: subclavian artery, vein, and nerve cords.

Technique: place a linear array ultrasound probe in a lateral position at the deltopectoral triangle to obtain a SAX view of the plexus. The subclavian artery and vein, and the medial and lateral cords of the plexus, should be visible. To visualize the posterior cord (and the pleura), it may be necessary to tilt the probe obliquely. To anaesthetize each cord individually, insert the needle either superior or inferior to the probe, using an IP approach. Confirm needle placement with a test dose of anaesthetic. Deposit 5–6 mL of anaesthetic around each cord. A ring of anaesthetic should be visible around each cord. Alternatively, the plexus may be anaesthetized without identifying and anaesthetizing each individual cord. Visualize the subclavian artery, and aim to deposit a U-shaped bolus superior, posterior, and inferior to the artery. The maximum total volume injected is 20 mL.

Needle: 21–22 G, 9 cm, Stimuplex®.

Local anaesthetic: 1.5–2% lignocaine, 0.75–1% ropivacaine, or a 1:1 mixture of 2% lignocaine and 1% ropivacaine.

Comments: the skin and pectoralis major muscle can be infiltrated with anaesthetic prior to injection to increase patient comfort. It is not uncommon to see the posterior cord fused with another cord, most commonly the medial cord. Abducting the arm 110° and externally rotating the shoulder bring the brachial plexus more superficial and pleura anterior, thus care is required with needle insertion. Deposition of a U-shaped bolus under the subclavian artery is quicker and easier to perform than identifying and anaesthetizing each cord of the plexus individually. The target point for single injection technique or catheter placement is cephaloposterior to the artery. Local anaesthetic will displace the subclavian artery anteriorly if the correct U-shaped deposit is achieved. For continuous catheter techniques, place the catheter in the cephaloposterior quadrant behind the subclavian artery, adjacent to the posterior cord. In this quandrant, all three cords are in close proximity.

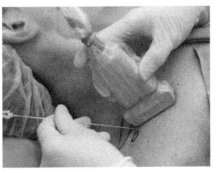

FIGURE 3.23 Insert the needle superior to the probe, using an IP approach.

FIGURE 3.24 SAX view of the infraclavicular.

a   Pectoralis major
b   Pectoralis minor
c   Subclavian a.
d   Subclavian v.
e   Brachial plexus

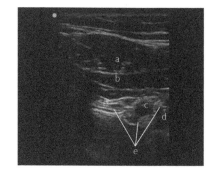

FIGURE 3.25 SAX view of the infraclavicular CFD.

a   Subclavian v. (oblique view)

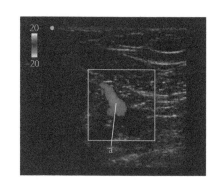

FIGURE 3.26

1   Needle path
2   Pectoralis major m.
3   Pectoralis minor m.
4   Subclavian a.
5   U-shaped deposit of local anaesthetic

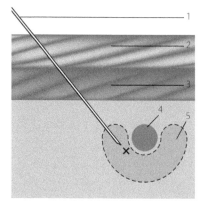

Infraclavicular plexus block: lateral approach

COMPLEXITY: ●●○

Indications
- Anaesthesia and analgesia for the upper and lower arm, and hand surgery
- Analgesia for physiotherapeutic treatment
- Treatment of pain syndrome
- Sympathicolysis.

Specific contraindications
- Thorax deformity
- Foreign bodies in the needle insertion area (e.g. pacemaker)
- Clavicular malunion.

Side effects and complications
- Intravascular injection
- Pneumothorax.

See Figures 3.27 and 3.28.

Single injection technique[6]

Patient position: supine, with the patient's head turned away from the side to be blocked and arm abducted 90° and elevated 30°.

Landmarks: jugular notch, acromion (ventral process), and axillary artery.

Technique: palpate the jugular notch and the ventral process of the acromion. Insert the needle approximately 1 cm caudad to the clavicle at the midpoint between these landmarks. Direct the needle laterally at a 45–60° angle towards the most proximal point where the axillary artery can still be palpated in the axilla. Advance the needle 3–8 cm. Stimulation at this depth with a current of 0.2–0.3 mA/0.1 ms should elicit flexion of the hand or fingers (median nerve). Inject 30 mL of anaesthetic slowly.

Needle: 22 G, 6–10 cm, insulated.

Local anaesthetic: 1% lignocaine (30–40 mL), 0.5% bupivacaine, or 0.75% ropivacaine.

Comments: the risk of pneumothorax is low, as the needle is inserted and directed laterally.

FIGURE 3.27

1   Suprascapular n.
2   Deltoid m.
3   Brachial plexus
    (infraclavicular)
4   Pectoral n.
5   Subclavian a.
6   Pectoralis major m.

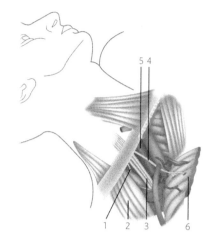

FIGURE 3.28 Direct the needle towards the most proximal point of the axillary artery at a 45–60° angle.

a   Axillary a.
b   Needle insertion site

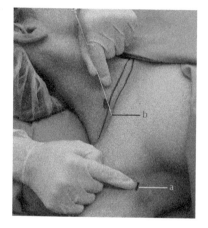

Suprascapular nerve block

COMPLEXITY: ✪✪✪

Indications

- Anaesthesia supplementary to incomplete interscalene plexus block
- Analgesia of shoulder conditions (adhesive capsulitis, arthritis, rupture of the rotator cuff)
- Diagnostic for shoulder pain of unclear origin.

See Figures 3.29 and 3.30.

Single injection technique[4]

Patient position: sitting, with the hand of the shoulder to be blocked placed on the opposing shoulder.

Landmarks: acromion (lateral posterior portion) and scapula (medial border).

Technique: palpate the lateral posterior portion of the acromion and the medial border of the scapula. Draw a line to connect these two landmarks, and mark its midpoint. Insert the needle 2 cm cephalad and 2 cm lateral from the midpoint. Direct the needle laterocaudadly and slightly ventral towards the head of the humerus at an angle of approximately 30°. Advance the needle to a depth of 3–5 cm where stimulation elicits motor responses in the supraspinatus and infraspinatus muscles. Inject 10–15 mL of anaesthetic slowly.

Needle: 22 G, 6–8 cm, insulated.

Local anaesthetic: 1% lignocaine, 0.5% bupivacaine, or 0.75% ropivacaine.

Comments: the risk of pneumothorax is limited if recommended guidelines are followed. Although extremely rare, aspirate to avoid intravascular injection in the suprascapular artery. If nerve stimulation is unsuccessful in locating the nerve, anaesthetic may be injected into the supraspinous groove, as detected by bony contact.

FIGURE 3.29

1 Supraspinatus m.
2 Infraspinatus m.
3 Trapezius m.
4 Suprascapular a.
5 Transverse scapular ligament
6 Suprascapular n.
7 Suprascapular n. (articular branches)
8 Deltoid m.

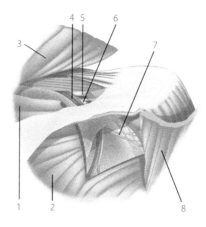

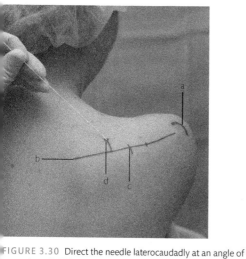

FIGURE 3.30 Direct the needle laterocaudadly at an angle of approximately 30°.

a Acromion (lateral posterior portion)
b Scapula (medial border)
c Midpoint between the acromion (lateral posterior portion) and the scapula (medial border)
d Needle insertion site

Axillary plexus block

COMPLEXITY: ✪✪✪

Indications
- Anaesthesia and analgesia for the distal upper arm, forearm, and hand surgery
- Physiotherapy
- Pain syndrome
- Sympathicolysis.

See Figures 3.31 and 3.32.

Single injection technique

Patient position: supine, with head facing away from the side of the block. Abduct the arm to be blocked 90° and rotate externally, and flex elbow 90°.

Landmarks: axillary artery and coracobrachialis muscle.

Technique: palpate the axillary artery and coracobrachialis muscle. Insert the needle between these two landmarks. Direct the needle proximally and parallel to the artery at a 30–45° angle to the skin. When the needle penetrates the neurovascular sheath (although unreliable, a click or pop may be felt), lower the distal end and advance 1–2 cm. Effortless needle advancement indicates correct needle placement and can be confirmed by nerve stimulation (which improves the success of this block when performed by inexperienced anaesthetists). Inject 40 mL of anaesthetic slowly.

Needle: 18 G, 4 cm, short bevel (45°), insulated.

Local anaesthetic: 1.5% lignocaine, 0.25–0.5% bupivacaine, or 0.75% ropivacaine.

Comments: a supplementary radial and musculocutaneous nerve block may be required if anaesthesia of the radial nerve distribution is insufficient.

Continuous catheter technique

Technique: locate the nerve, as described above. Perform continuous catheter technique, as described under Catheter technique for continuous infusions.

Equipment: StimuCath™, or Plexolong or Contiplex® (19.5 G, 3–6 cm, insulated Tuohy needle and wire-stiffened 20 G catheter).

Local anaesthetic: 0.2% ropivacaine.

FIGURE 3.31

1 Coracobrachialis m.

2 Radial n.

3 Medial antebrachial cutaneous n. (posterior to the basilic v.)

4 Ulnar n.

5 Brachial a.

6 Median n.

7 Musculocutaneous n.

8 Pectoralis major m.

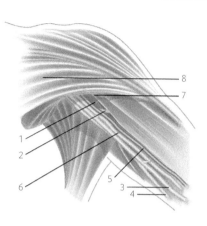

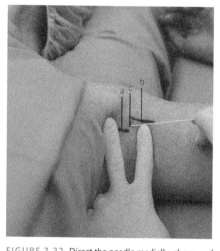

FIGURE 3.32 Direct the needle medially, above and parallel to the axillary artery at a 30–45° angle to the skin.

a Axillary a.

b Coracobrachialis m.

c Needle insertion site

Axillary plexus block

COMPLEXITY: ●●○
See Figures 3.33, 3.34, and 3.35.

Ultrasound-guided technique

Patient position: supine, with head facing away from the side of the block. Abduct the arm to be blocked 90° and rotate externally, and flex elbow 90°.

Landmarks: surface: pectoralis major muscle; sonoanatomical: axillary artery.

Technique: to obtain a SAX view of the axillary plexus, place the ultrasound probe perpendicular to the skin, in line with the pectoralis major muscle. Move the probe distally. Minimal pressure on the probe will ensure visualization of the multiple veins surrounding the axillary artery. Typically, the median nerve is located superoanteriorly, the ulnar nerve inferoposteriorly, and the radial nerve posteriorly to the axillary artery. The musculocutaneous nerve is seen either within the coracobrachialis muscle or, more commonly, in a fascial plane between the biceps brachii and coracobrachialis muscles. Insert the needle, using an IP approach. Confirm needle placement with a test dose of anaesthetic. Inject 5 mL of anaesthetic around each nerve.

Needle: 21 G, 4 cm, Stimuplex®.

Local anaesthetic: 1.5–2% lignocaine, 0.75–1% ropivacaine, or a 1:1 mixture of 2% lignocaine and 1% ropivacaine.

Comments: the location of the median, radial, and ulnar nerves around the axillary artery varies significantly from patient to patient. Visualizing their location by ultrasound allows direct deposition of anaesthetic on each nerve and ensures a higher success rate, compared with the single-shot, high-volume approach.

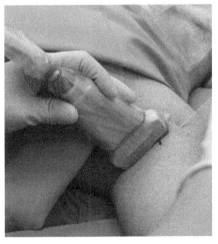

FIGURE 3.33 Insert the needle, using an IP approach.

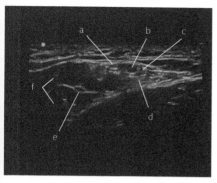

FIGURE 3.34 SAX view of the axilla.

a   Median n.   d   Radial n.
b   Axillary a.   e   Musculocutaneous n.
c   Ulnar n.   f   Biceps m.

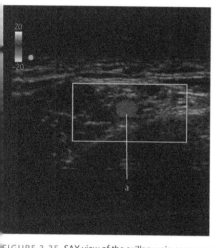

FIGURE 3.35 SAX view of the axillary vein compressed CFD.

a   Axillary a.

Supplementary blocks for the upper limb

COMPLEXITY: ★★★

An incomplete brachial plexus block may be supplemented by additional nerve blocks in the upper arm or in the mid-forearm. Ultrasound guidance is recommended, as it avoids dependence on palpable surface landmarks, ensures needle trajectories are directed away from vascular structures, improves accuracy, and allows local anaesthetic deposition distant from the cubital tunnel.

Indications

• Incomplete brachial plexus block.

See Figures 3.36, 3.37, and 3.38.

Ultrasound-guided technique: radial nerve block

Patient position: supine, with arm placed over the abdomen.

Landmarks: surface: brachial artery; sonoanatomical: brachial artery.

Technique: place a linear 38 mm, high-frequency 10–15 MHz transducer on the lateral aspect of the distal third of the upper arm. Locate the radial nerve within the spiral groove, adjacent to the humerus bone, and deep to the triceps muscle. Scanning in a cephalad direction, the nerve moves away from the humerus and travels laterally towards the lateral condyle. The profunda brachii artery is often seen accompanying the nerve, assisting in its identification. Inject 2–5 mL of local anaesthetic around the radial nerve.

Needle: 22 G, 5 cm.

Local anaesthetic: 0.75% ropivacaine.

FIGURE 3.36

1. Musculocutaneous n.
2. Median n.
3. Ulnar n.
4. Radial n.

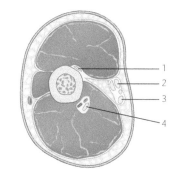

FIGURE 3.37
Radial nerve
block at the spiral
groove; insert the
needle, using an IP
approach.

a. Shoulder
b. Elbow

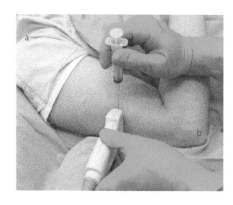

FIGURE 3.38 SAX
view of the radial
spiral groove.

a. Radial n.
b. Humerus

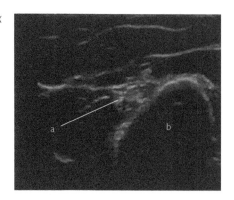

Supplementary blocks for the upper limb

COMPLEXITY: ● ○ ○
See Figures 3.39, 3.40, 3.41, and 3.42.

Ultrasound-guided technique: ulnar nerve block

Patient position: supine, arm rotated and flexed to expose the medial aspect of the forearm.

Landmarks: surface: ulnar artery; sonoanatomical: ulnar artery.

Technique: the ulnar nerve can be identified distally at the wrist by its association with the ulnar artery. Once identified, scan proximally until the nerve moves away from the artery—in the mid-forearm—and block at this level to minimize the risk of accidental arterial injection. Alternatively, trace the ulnar nerve from the cubital tunnel distally into the mid-forearm. Inject 2–5 mL of local anaesthetic, aiming to achieve circumferential spread around the ulnar nerve.

Needle: 25 G, hypodermic.

Local anaesthetic: 0.75% ropivacaine.

Ultrasound-guided technique: median nerve block

Patient position: supine, with arm supinated at the antecubital fossa.

Landmarks: surface: brachial artery; sonoanatomical: brachial artery.

Technique: the median nerve lies immediately deep to the bicipital aponeurosis, medial to the pulsatile brachial artery. The median nerve block is performed in the proximal third of the forearm, choosing a needle trajectory away from the brachial artery, either OOP or IP. Block the medial nerve in the mid-forearm where it is easily visualized and separated from other structures. A median nerve block, in combination with an ulnar nerve block, is useful for hand surgery involving the palm of the hand. Inject 2–5 mL of local anaesthetic, aiming to achieve circumferential spread around the median nerve.

Needle: 25 G, hypodermic.

Local anaesthetic: 0.75% ropivacaine.

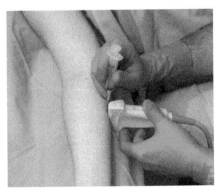

FIGURE 3.39 Ulnar nerve block. Insert the needle, using an IP approach.

FIGURE 3.40 SAX
view of the
ulnar nerve.

a   Ulnar n.
b   Tendon
c   Ulnar a.

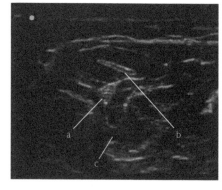

FIGURE 3.41
Median nerve
block. Insert the
needle, using an IP
approach.

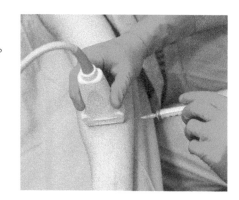

FIGURE 3.42 SAX
view of the
median nerve.

a   Median n.

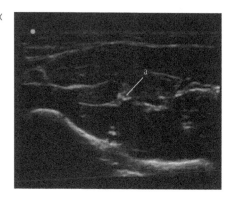

Wrist blocks

COMPLEXITY: ⬤○○

This is a basic, non-ultrasound block. If ultrasound is used, the medial, radial, and ulnar nerves should be approached, using the ultrasound-guided techniques described under Supplementary blocks for the upper limb.

Indications
- Analgesia and anaesthesia for hand surgery
- Management of fractured metacarpals and lacerated hands
- Supplementation of incomplete brachial block.

Specific contraindications
- History of nerve entrapment syndromes.

See Figures 3.43, 3.44, and 3.45.

Technique

Median nerve

Patient position: arm is stretched laterally and externally rotated, and hand supine.

Landmarks: palmaris longus muscle tendon and palmar crease.

Technique: insert the needle at the palmar crease on the ulnar side of the tendon of the palmaris longus muscle, and direct towards the ulna (away from the nerve). Ask the patient to move their fingers, and adjust the needle to ensure that it is not inserted into a tendon. Inject 4–5 mL of anaesthetic slowly. A diffuse swelling indicates deposition of anaesthetic deep to the flexor retinaculum and correct needle placement. A discrete bleb indicates superficial needle placement, resulting in an ineffective block. Anaesthesia can be achieved, albeit slowly, by manually pushing the bleb in a radial direction to spread the anaesthetic across to the nerve.

Needle: 25 G, 1 cm.

Local anaesthetic: 1% lignocaine, 0.5% bupivacaine, or 0.75% ropivacaine.

Comments: in the classic approach, the needle is placed between the tendons of the palmaris longus muscle and the flexor carpi ulnaris muscle.

Ulnar nerve

Patient position: arm is stretched laterally and externally rotated, and hand supine.

Landmark: flexor carpi ulnaris muscle tendon.

Technique: palpate the tendon of the flexor carpi ulnaris muscle. Insert the needle posterolaterally, and direct horizontally. Withdraw the needle and redirect if paraesthesiae is elicited. Inject 3–5 mL of anaesthetic slowly.

Needle: 27 G, 1 cm.

Local anaesthetic: 1% lignocaine, 0.5% bupivacaine, or 0.75% ropivacaine.

Comments: this approach avoids the artery and allows the anaesthetic to 'float' up from behind the tendon. In the classic approach, the anaesthetic is injected medial to the artery at the dorsum of the wrist. The classic approach is associated with greater neuropraxia.

FIGURE 3.43

1 Pisiform bone
2 Ulnar n.
3 Ulnar a.
4 Flexor carpi ulnaris m. tendon
5 Palmaris m. longus tendon
6 Flexor carpi radialis m. tendon
7 Median n.
8 Radial a.

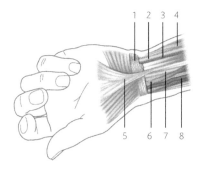

FIGURE 3.44 To block the median nerve, insert the needle at the palmar crease on the ulnar side of the palmaris longus m. tendon.

a Needle insertion site

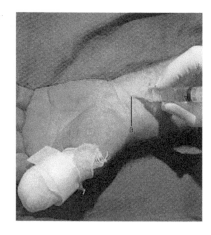

FIGURE 3.45 To block the ulnar nerve, insert the needle posterolaterally to the flexor carpi ulnaris m. tendon.

a Needle insertion site

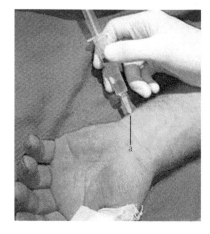

Wrist blocks

COMPLEXITY: ✪✪✪
See Figures 3.46 and 3.47.

Technique

Radial nerve

Patient position: arm is stretched laterally, and hand supine.

Technique: insert the needle on the radial side of the wrist, 3–5 cm proximal to the joint, and infiltrate 10 mL of anaesthetic subcutaneously.

Needle: 22–24 G, 1 cm.

Local anaesthetic: 1% lignocaine, 0.5% bupivacaine, or 0.75% ropivacaine.

FIGURE 3.46

1 Radial
   n. (superficial
   branches)

2 Radial a.

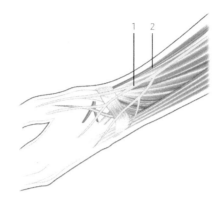

FIGURE 3.47 To
block the radial
nerve, insert the
needle on the radial
side of wrist.

a Needle
   insertion site

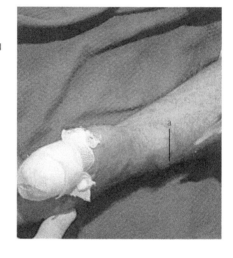

References

1 Perlas A and Chan V. Ultrasound-assisted nerve blocks.
New York: New York School of Regional Anaesthesia. Viewed 19
October 2009, <http://www.nysora.com/peripheral_nerve_blocks/
ultrasound-guided_techniques/3063-ultrasound_assisted_nerve_blocks.
html>.
2 Seltzer J (1977). Hoarseness and Horner's syndrome after interscalene
brachial plexus block. *Anesth Analg* **56**, 585-6.
3 Urmey W and McDonald M (1992). Hemidiaphragmatic paresis during
interscalene brachial plexus block: effects on pulmonary function and chest
mechanics. *Anesth Analg* **74**, 352-7.
4 Meier G and Büttner J (2005). *Regional anaesthesia. Pocket compendium of
peripheral nerve blocks.* 3rd edn. Munich: Acris Publishing Company.
5 Marhofer P, Greher M, Kapral S (2005). Ultrasound guidance in regional
anaesthesia. *Br J Anaesth* **94**, 7-17.
6 Borgeat A, Ekatodramis G, Dumont C (2001). An evaluation of the
infraclavicular block via a modified approach of the Raj technique. *Anesth
Analg* **95**, 436-41.

Anatomy of the lumbosacral plexus

Lumbar plexus

The lumbar plexus is formed by the ventral rami of the L1–L4 spinal nerves. Nerves of the lower extremities relevant for anaesthesia include the femoral nerve and its terminal branch, the saphenous nerve, the lateral femoral cutaneous nerve, and the obturator nerve.

The femoral nerve is the largest branch of the lumbar plexus and arises from the second, third, and fourth lumbar nerves. It supplies the anterior and medial thigh, femur, patella, and majority of the knee joint, as well as the cutaneous strip along the medial calf to the medial malleous and medial instep. See Figure 4.1.

Sacral plexus

The sacral plexus is formed by the ventral rami of the L4 and L5 spinal nerves (lumbosacral trunk) and S1–S3. Nerves of the lower extremities relevant to anaesthesia include the sciatic nerve and its terminal branches, the common peroneal nerve and tibial nerve, and the posterior femoral cutaneous nerve. See Figure 4.2.

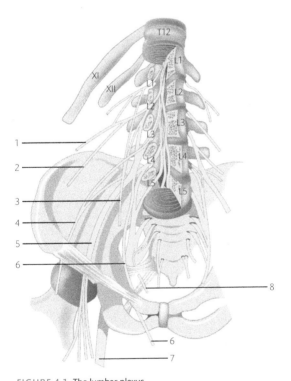

FIGURE 4.1 The lumbar plexus.

1	Iliohypogastric n.	5	Femoral n.
2	Ilioinguinal n.	6	Obturator n.
3	Genitofemoral n.	7	Sciatic n.
4	Lateral femoral cutaneous n.	8	Pudendal n.

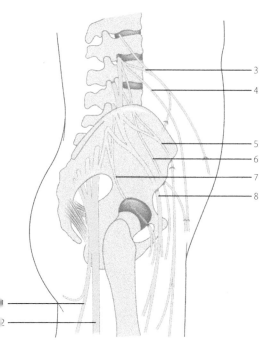

FIGURE 4.2 The sacral plexus.

1	Posterior femoral cutaneous n.	5	Lateral femoral cutaneous n.
2	Sciatic n.	6	Genitofemoral n.
3	Iliohypogastric n.	7	Obturator n.
4	Ilioinguinal n.	8	Femoral n.

Sensory supply of the lower extremities

See Figure 4.3.

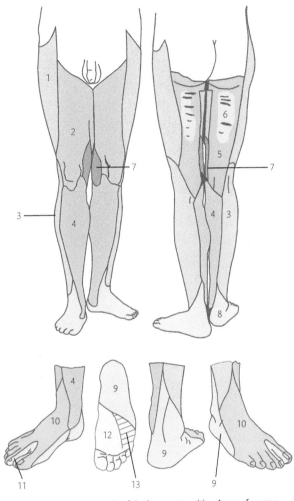

FIGURE 4.3 Sensory supply of the lower extremities. Areas of sensory distribution: ● Femoral n. and its branches ● Sciatic n. and its branches ● Lateral femoral cutaneous n. ● Obturator n.

1	Lateral femoral cutaneous n.	8	Posterior tibial n.
2	Femoral n.	9	Sural n.
3	Peroneal n.	10	Superficial peroneal n.
4	Saphenous n.	11	Deep peroneal n.
5	Sciatic n.	12	Medial plantar n.
6	Posterior femoral cuta neous n.	13	Lateral plantar n. (tibial n.)
7	Obturator n.		

Sensory supply of the bony structure

See Figure 4.4.

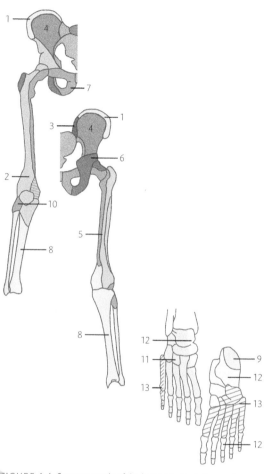

FIGURE 4.4 Sensory supply of the bony structure. Areas of sensory distribution: ● Femoral n. and its branches ● Sciatic n. and its branches ● Obturator n. (variable innervation).

1 Collateral branch of femoral n.	8 Tibial and posterior tibial nerves
2 Femoral n.	9 Sural n.
3 Superior gluteal n.	10 Common peroneal n.
4 Inferior gluteal n.	11 Deep peroneal n.
5 Sciatic n.	12 Medial plantar n.
6 Sacral nerves	13 Lateral plantar n.
7 Obturator n.	

Motor response

See Figure 4.5.

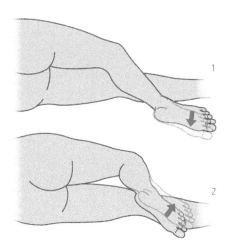

FIGURE 4.5 Motor response.

1 Tibial n.: plantarflexion (foot inversion)
2 Peroneal n.: dorsiflexion (foot eversion)

Scanning tips for the lower extremities

Lumbosacral plexus

Innervation to the lower extremity is provided by the lumbosacral plexus. Imaging of the lumbosacral plexus and its proximal branches may be difficult due to the depth of these structures.[1]

Lumbar plexus

The patient should be positioned either prone, with a pillow under the abdomen to reduce lumbar lordosis, lateral, or sitting. Use a curved 4–5 MHz probe to image the paravertebral region. Identify the lumbar transverse processes approximately 3 cm from the midline by positioning the probe longitudinally in a parasagittal plane. Turn the transducer 90° into the transverse axial plane, positioning it between two transverse processes to minimize the interference to the ultrasound beam. Deep to the subcutaneous plane, identify the erector spinae muscle immediately lateral to the spinous process and, more laterally, the smaller quadratus lumborum. Anterior to these two muscles, the psoas muscle lies adjacent to the vertebral bodies and intervertebral discs. The lumbar plexus is usually found between the anterior two-thirds and the posterior third of the psoas muscle. The plexus may be difficult to identify with ultrasound alone; adjuvant use of nerve stimulation is recommended. Administer local anaesthetic in the plexus with this technique. Avoid inadvertent needle trauma to the kidney by identification of the inferior pole of the kidney, as low as L3–L4.[1]

See Figures 4.6, 4.7, and 4.8 for a demonstration of this technique.

Femoral nerve—lumbar/inguinal

The lumbar plexus has three main terminal branches, the femoral, obturator, and lateral femoral cutaneous nerves. The largest branch is the femoral nerve, derived from L2–L4. Use a linear 10–15 MHz transducer, placed over the inguinal crease in the transverse axial plane, to identify the hyperechoic oval or triangular-shaped femoral nerve lateral to the femoral vessels. The femoral nerve overlies the iliopectineal arch, overlying the groove between the iliac and psoas muscles, and, for a short distance, may be imaged distally until it divides into small terminal branches, indistinguishable sonographically from the surrounding tissue. The saphenous nerve may be imaged next to the femoral vessels in the mid- to distal thigh.[1]

See Figure 4.9.

Sciatic nerve—proximal/anterior mid-thigh/distal

The lumbosacral plexus is the origin of the sciatic nerve, which enters the gluteal region between two muscle planes through the greater sciatic foramen. The obturator internus and inferior gemellus form the anterior muscle plane, while the more superficial gluteus maximus muscle forms the posterior plane. The depth of the sciatic nerve in the gluteal region makes it difficult to identify; it lies more superficial in the subgluteal region.[1]

Position the patient semi-prone, with the limb to be blocked uppermost. Use a curved 2–7 MHz transducer to obtain a transverse view of the sciatic nerve. The greater trochanter of the femur is identified laterally and the ischial tuberosity medially; the sciatic nerve lies approximately in the midpoint of a line between both landmarks. Frequently, the appearance of the sciatic nerve is hyperechoic and elliptical, deep to the distal gluteus maximus muscle and lateral to the biceps femoris muscle. The aponeurosis of the surrounding muscles surrounds the sciatic nerve as a well-defined border.[1]

A 7–15 MHz linear probe may be used to image the sciatic nerve more caudally to the popliteal fossa. Here, the sciatic nerve often appears round and hyperechoic, lying posterior to the femur, lateral and superficial to the popliteal artery, and anterior to the semitendinous and semimembranous muscles medially and the biceps femoris muscle laterally, before dividing into the peroneal and tibial nerves. Moving distally, the peroneal nerve may be followed to the level of the head of the fibula.[1]

See Figures 4.10, 4.11, and 4.12.

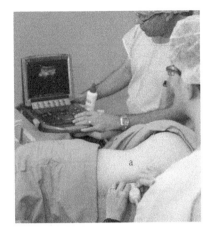

FIGURE 4.6 Scanning the lumbar plexus in the left lateral decubitus (semi-prone) position; position the curvilinear probe longitudinally in a parasagittal plane.

a   Right side of patient

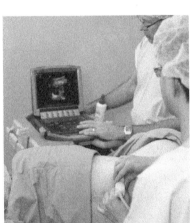

FIGURE 4.7 Next, position the curvilinear probe in the transverse axial plane between two transverse processes.

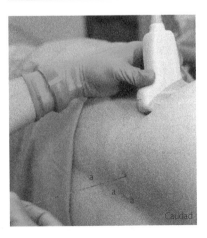

FIGURE 4.8 Relative positions of the probe and needle for an IP approach to the right lumbar plexus block.

a   Lumbar spine

FIGURE 4.9 Scanning the femoral nerve; use a linear transducer placed over the inguinal crease in the transverse axial plane.

a   Right thigh

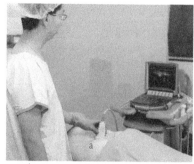

FIGURE 4.10 Scanning the proximal sciatic nerve, using a curvilinear probe.

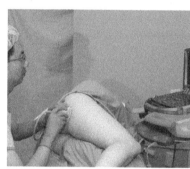

FIGURE 4.11 Scanning the distal sciatic nerve, using a linear probe.

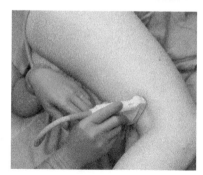

FIGURE 4.12 SAX view of the sciatic n. subgluteal.

a   Sciatic nerve
b   Gluteus maximus
c   Greater trochanter
d   Quadriceps femoris
e   Ischial tuberosity

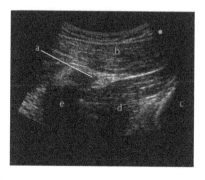

Psoas compartment (lumbar plexus) block

COMPLEXITY: ⊗⊗○

Indications
- Leg surgery when in combination with proximal sciatic nerve block
- Wound treatment in the ventral and lateral thigh regions
- Skin grafts in the upper thigh region
- Physiotherapy
- Analgesia (after hip or knee surgery).

Specific contraindications
- As per contraindications for neuroaxial block.

Side effects and complications
- Spinal anaesthesia
- Spread of anaesthetic to the epidural space, causing an epidural-like block
- Haematoma.

See Figures 4.13 and 4.14.

Technique
Patient position: lateral with legs flexed, the operative leg uppermost, and the back kyphotic.

Landmarks: intercristal line, ischial tuberosity (IT), and posterior superior iliac spine (PSIS).

Technique: palpate the iliac crests, and mark the intercristal line. Locate the projection of the IT posteriorly and the PSIS. Draw a line connecting these two landmarks, and extend it to intersect the intercristal line. Insert the needle at right angles to all surfaces. The needle may contact the transverse process of L5. If so, withdraw the needle 1–3 cm, and redirect more cephalad. The plexus will be 10–15 mm deeper. Contraction of the quadratus femoris muscle at a stimulating current of 0.3 mA/0.1 ms indicates correct needle placement. Inject a test dose to preclude an intraspinal needle position prior to injecting 30 mL of anaesthetic slowly.

Needle: 22 G, 15 cm, insulated, Stimuplex®.

Local anaesthetic: 1% lignocaine or 0.75% ropivacaine (20–30 mL).

Comments: infiltration is recommended prior to needle insertion. Anaesthetic injected at the level of the L3 spinous process does not improve the quality of anaesthesia and carries a risk of causing a subcapsular haematoma of the kidney. Injection into the peritoneal cavity may occur when the needle depth is very deep. A complete block of the sacral plexus at this level is not possible, even with higher volumes of anaesthetic.

Continuous catheter technique
Technique: locate the nerve, as described in the previous section. Perform the continuous catheter technique, as described under Catheter technique for continuous infusions.

Equipment: StimuCath™, or Plexolong or Contiplex® (19.5 G, 15 cm, insulated Tuohy needle and 20 G catheter).

Local anaesthetic: 0.2% ropivacaine.

FIGURE 4.13

1 Lumbar plexus
2 Psoas major m.
3 Fascia iliaca
4 Transverse process
   (costal process)
5 Erector spinae m.
6 Needle direction

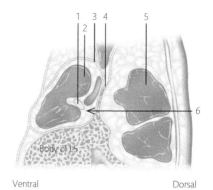

Ventral   Dorsal

FIGURE 4.14

a Intercristal line
b Ischial tuberosity
c Posterior superior
   iliac spine
d Needle insertion site

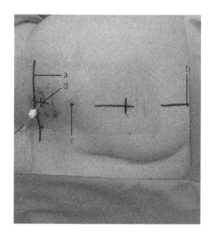

Psoas compartment (lumbar plexus) block

COMPLEXITY: ✪✪✪
See Figures 4.15 to 4.19.

Ultrasound-guided technique

Patient position: lateral with legs flexed, the operative leg uppermost, and the back kyphotic.

Landmarks: surface: L2–L5 spinous processes; sonoanatomical: psoas major, quadratus lumborum, and erector spinae muscles.

Technique: place a 2–5 MHz curved-array ultrasound probe along the L2–L5 spinous processes, and locate the L3 and L4 vertebra in a longitudinal view. Rotate the probe into a transverse view, and visualize the transverse process of L4, the psoas major, the quadratus lumborum, and the erector spinae muscles. Using the frequency and gain controls, optimize the sonoanatomy image and ensure the psoas major, the quadratus lumborum, and the erector spinae muscles are clearly delineated. Identify the junction of the posterior third and anterior two-thirds of the psoas major muscle. This is the reference point for needle advancement. Insert the needle 4–5 cm lateral to the spinous process and medial to the probe, and perpendicular to the skin, using an IP approach. Advance the needle to the reference point, and inject 30 mL of anaesthetic slowly.

Needle: 22 G, 12 cm, insulated, Tuohy.

Local anaesthetic: 1.5–2% lignocaine, 0.75–1% ropivacaine, or a 1:1 mixture of 2% lignocaine and 1% ropivacaine.

Comments: a curved-array probe at lower frequencies provides appropriate tissue penetration and image size but less spatial resolution. This may create difficulty and cause poor differentiation between peripheral nerves and tendon fibres within the psoas major muscle. As it is often not possible to visualize the lumbar plexus within the psoas major muscle, neurostimulation is a useful adjunct to ultrasound for this block. The patient may also be positioned sitting, with the lumbar region kyphotic (as shown in Figures 4.15 and 4.18).

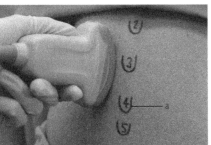

FIGURE 4.15
Ultrasound probe position for a longitudinal SAX view of the psoas compartment.

a   L4 spinous process

FIGURE 4.16
Longitudinal SAX view of
the psoas muscle.

a   Lumbosacral plexus

b   Psoas m.

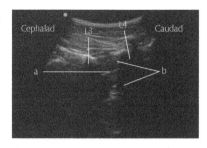

FIGURE 4.17
Longitudinal SAX view
of the psoas muscle and
kidney.

a   Erector spinae m.

b   Psoas m.

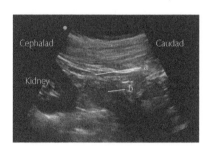

FIGURE 4.18
Transverse SAX
view of the psoas
compartment.

a   Psoas major m.

b   Erector spinae m.

c   Quadratus
    lumborum m.
    L4 transverse process

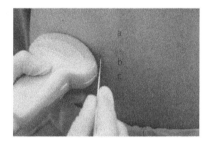

FIGURE 4.19
Transverse SAX view of
the psoas.

a   Psoas m.

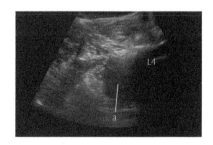

Femoral nerve block

COMPLEXITY: ●●●

In this technique, the needle is inserted a few centimetres below, rather than at, the level of the inguinal ligament. The '3-in-1 block',[2] which blocks the femoral, lateral femoral cutaneous, and obturator nerves, is only truly a '3-in-1 block' one-third of the time. Successful blockade of the obturator nerve with this technique is low. In addition, the lateral femoral cutaneous nerve is blocked in only 50% of these blocks performed if a large volume of anaesthetic is injected, presumably a result of the lateral spread of anaesthetic.[3]

Indications

- Surgery of the anterior thigh and knee, and quadriceps tendon repair
- Post-operative analgesia after femur or knee surgery, knee arthroplasty, anterior cruciate ligament or femoral fracture repair.

See Figures 4.20, 4.21, and 4.22.

Technique

Patient position: supine, with both legs extended. Place a pillow underneath the hips of obese patients to facilitate palpation of the femoral artery.

Landmarks: inguinal ligament and femoral artery pulse.

Technique: infiltrate the needle insertion area subcutaneously. Palpate the inguinal ligament and the pulse of the femoral artery. Standing to the side of the patient, with one hand palpating the femoral artery, insert the needle at the lateral border of the artery, and advance in a sagittal and slightly cephalad plane. A visible or palpable twitch of the quadratus femoris muscle at 0.2–0.5 mA/0.1 ms, reduced from 1.0 mA/0.1 ms, indicates correct needle placement. If twitching occurs in the sartorius muscle only, redirect the needle laterally, and advance several millimetres deeper. Inject 20 mL of anaesthetic slowly.

Needle: skin infiltration: 25 G, 3 cm; injection: 25 G, 5 cm, short bevel, insulated.

Local anaesthetic: 1.5% lignocaine with adrenaline 1:200 000, 0.5% bupivacaine, or 0.75% ropivacaine.

Comments: always confirm correct needle placement with quadratus femoris muscle twitching, as stimulation of the sartorius muscle can be obtained in or outside of the sheath of the femoral nerve. The nerve to the sartorius muscle appears medial to, and travels over, the femoral nerve, entering the sartorius muscle laterally. If the sartorius muscle is stimulated, redirect the needle medially, laterally, or deeper.

Continuous catheter technique

Technique: locate the nerve, as described previously. Perform the continuous catheter technique, as described under Catheter technique for continuous infusions.

Equipment: StimuCath™, or Plexolong or Contiplex® (19.5 G, 3–6 cm, insulated Tuohy needle and 20 G catheter).

Local anaesthetic: 0.25% bupivacaine or 0.2% ropivacaine.

Comments: care should be taken to avoid medial insertion of the needle and the consequent puncture of the femoral artery.

FIGURE 4.20

a   Inguinal ligament
b   Femoral a.

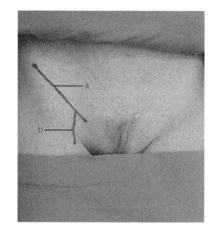

FIGURE 4.21

1   Fascia lata
2   Femoral n.
3   Femoral a.
4   Femoral v.
5   Femoral sheath
6   Fascia iliaca
7   Ilioacus m.
8   Pectineus m.

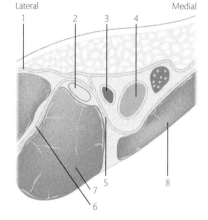

FIGURE 4.22 Insert and direct the needle in a sagittal and slightly cephalad plane.

a   Needle insertion site

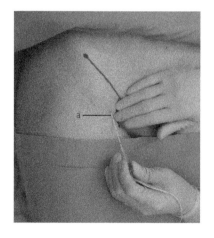

Femoral nerve block

COMPLEXITY: ✪ ✪ ✪
See Figures 4.23 to 4.27.

Ultrasound-guided technique

Patient position: supine.

Landmarks: surface: inguinal ligament; sonoanatomical: femoral vein and femoral artery. In most patients, the femoral artery is a useful orientation marker, as it is located medial to the femoral nerve.

Technique: palpate the inguinal ligament. Place a high-frequency (>7 MHz) linear-array ultrasound probe on, and in line with, the inguinal ligament. From medial to lateral, the femoral vein, femoral artery, and femoral nerve should be visible below the iliopectineal fascia. The needle can be inserted, using an IP or OOP approach. For the OOP approach, position the probe so that the femoral nerve is centre of the screen, as it correlates well with the midpoint of the lateral surface of the probe. This optimizes needle insertion and femoral nerve visualization. For the IP approach, insert the needle on the lateral edge of the probe. In both approaches, advance the needle towards the femoral nerve. Visualize the needle tip penetrating the iliopectineal fascia to ensure positioning of the needle within the femoral canal. Confirm needle placement with a test dose of anaesthetic. Inject 20 mL of anaesthetic, repositioning the needle while injecting to optimize the spread of anaesthetic. Hypoechoic expansion of fluid will occur and is easily visualized and will be contained wholly under the iliopectineal fascia.

Needle: 20 or 21 G, Stimuplex®.

Local anaesthetic: 1.5–2% lignocaine, 0.75–1% ropivacaine, or a 1:1 mixture of 2% lignocaine and 1% ropivacaine.

Comments: as the sonoanatomy and course of the femoral nerve vary among patients, scan above and below the inguinal ligament to identify variations in vascular structures and identify the course of the femoral nerve. This will assist in selecting the most appropriate needle insertion site and direction for approaching the femoral nerve. A Tuohy needle will assist cephalad catheter placement for continuous injection. In some patients, the nerve may be difficult to identify, and the use of a nerve stimulator can be helpful. The lateral circumflex femoral artery is usually a branch of the profunda femoris and may run under, or through, the femoral nerve. Use ultrasound to locate and identify this artery to minimize the risk of vascular puncture and injection. Preferential spread of local anaesthesia may also be adversely affected due to the division of the femoral nerve by the artery.

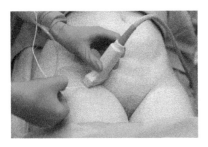

FIGURE 4.23 **Insert the needle, using an IP approach.**

FIGURE 4.24 SAX
view of the
femoral nerve.

a Femoral n.
b Iliacus m.
c Femoral a.
d Femoral v.

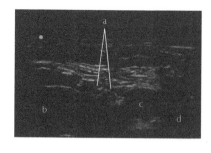

FIGURE 4.25 Oblique
SAX view of the
femoral nerve.

a Femoral n.
b Femoral a.
c Iliacus m.
d Quadriceps m.

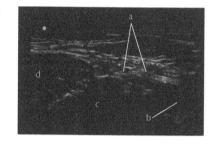

FIGURE 4.26 SAX
view of femoral nerve
with lateral circumflex
femoral artery.

a Lateral circumflex
   femoral a.
b Femoral v.
c Femoral a.
d Iliacus m.
e Femoral n. (divided)

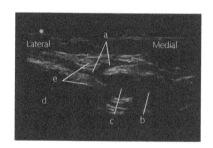

FIGURE 4.27 SAX
view of the lateral
femoral cutaneous
artery CFD.

a Lateral circumflex
   femoral a.
b Femoral a.

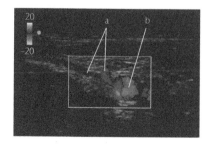

Lateral femoral cutaneous nerve block

COMPLEXITY: ⬤⬤◯

Indications

- Small skin grafts of the lateral aspect of the thigh
- Diagnostic tool for myalgia paraesthetica (neuralgia of the lateral cutaneous nerve of the thigh).

See Figures 4.28, 4.29, and 4.30.

Technique

Patient position: supine, with the anaesthetist at the patient's side.

Landmark: anterior superior iliac spine (ASIS).

Technique: insert the needle 2 cm medial and 2 cm caudad to the ASIS, and advance until a loss of resistance is felt as the needle passes through the fascia lata. Inject 10 mL of anaesthetic in a fanwise fashion, from medial and lateral, both above and below the fascia lata.

Needle: 22 G, 4 cm, short bevel.

Local anaesthetic: 2% lignocaine, 0.5% bupivacaine, or 0.75–1% ropivacaine.

Comment: fanwise injection is suggested, as the loss of resistance through the fascia lata is not consistent and perception of loss may vary among anaesthetists.

FIGURE 4.28

a Anterior superior iliac spine

b Needle insertion site

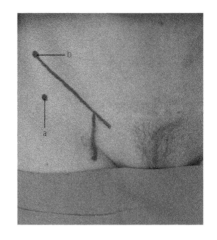

FIGURE 4.29

1 Anterior superior iliac spine

2 Lateral femoral cutaneous n.

3 Sartorius m.

4 Tensor fasciae latae m.

5 Femoral n.

6 Inguinal ligament

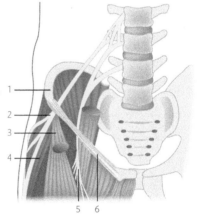

FIGURE 4.30 Direct the needle sagittally until a loss of resistance is felt.

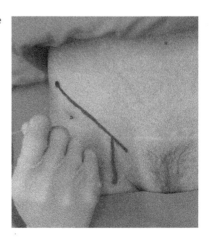

Fascia iliaca block

COMPLEXITY: ✪✪✪

The fascia iliaca block only reliably blocks the femoral and lateral femoral cutaneous nerves. This block has been previously described, using landmark techniques (Dalen's technique),[4] and relies on fascial clicks for correct needle depth. Ultrasound increases the ease, reliability, and safety of this block by allowing visualization of the needle, local anaesthetic spread, and fascial planes.

Indications

- Surgery in the region of the thigh and knee
- Anaesthesia in conjunction with sciatic nerve block
- It produces more reliable block of the lateral femoral cutaneous nerve of the thigh, compared to the 3-in-1 block.

See Figures 4.31 to 4.34.

Ultrasound-guided technique

Patient position: supine.

Landmarks: surface: ASIS, iliac bone; sonoanatomical: femoral vessels, iliacus muscle, fascia iliaca plane.

Technique: use a linear-array probe. For the inguinal technique, follow the fascia iliaca from the femoral vessels to the ASIS along the inguinal ligament. Perform the block, using either an IP or OOP approach. After confirmation of accurate needle positioning using 0.5–1.0 mL test bolus, hydrodissect the fascia iliaca using 20–30 mL of local anaesthetic.

For the suprainguinal technique, place the probe over, and perpendicular to, the inguinal ligament, scanning towards the xiphoid process. Locate the femoral artery medially and the anterior inferior iliac spine laterally, under the muscle belly of the iliacus. An IP approach is used, inserting the needle from the thigh and penetrating the fascia iliaca deep to the inguinal ligament. Confirm needle position with a test bolus, observing the spread of fluid between the iliacus muscle and the fascia iliaca, before hydrodissecting the plane using more local anaesthetic. A catheter may be inserted into the hydrodissected plane, if desired.

Needle: 21 G, 10 cm, short bevel, stimulating or Tuohy.

Local anaesthetic: 0.5–0.75% ropivacaine.

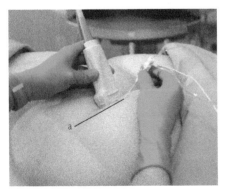

FIGURE 4.31
Insert the needle, using an OOP approach for the infrainguinal fascia iliaca block.

a Right inguinal crease

FIGURE 4.32
Fascia iliaca
infrainguinal
approach.

a Fascia iliaca
b Iliacus m.
c ASIS

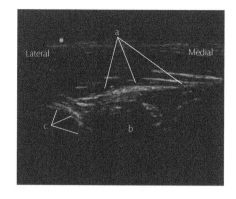

FIGURE 4.33
Insert the needle,
using an IP
approach for the
suprainguinal
fascia iliaca block.

a Right inguinal
   crease

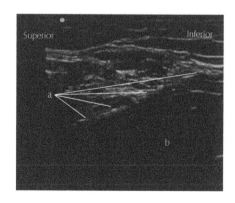

FIGURE 4.34
Fascia iliaca
suprainguinal
approach.

a Fascia iliaca
b Iliacus m.

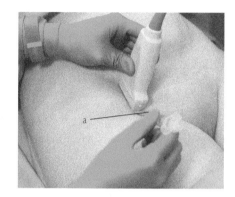

Obturator nerve block

COMPLEXITY: ✪✪✪

The anterior branch of the obturator nerve innervates the anterior adductor muscles, the hip joint, and, to a varying degree, a section of the skin on the inner surface of the thigh. The posterior branch of the obturator nerve innervates the deep adductor muscles and, to a varying degree, medial portions of the knee joint.

Indications

- Transurethral resection of tumours of the ipsilateral wall of the bladder
- Supplementary anaesthesia for incomplete lumbar plexus block
- Diagnosis/therapy for pain syndrome in the hip joint
- Adductor spasm.

See Figures 4.35, 4.36, and 4.37.

Technique

Patient position: supine, with leg abducted.

Landmark: adductor longus muscle (tendon).

Technique: palpate the proximal attachment point of the tendon of the adductor longus muscle. Insert the needle immediately ventral to the proximal attachment point of the tendon, and advance cephalad at a 45° angle to the longitudinal axis of the body and in a slightly dorsal direction. At a needle depth of 4–8 cm, contraction of the adductor muscles at a stimulating current of 0.3 mA/0.1 ms indicates proximity to the obturator nerve. Inject 10–15 mL of anaesthetic slowly.

Needle: 20 G, 10 cm, short bevel, insulated.

Local anaesthetic: 1% lignocaine, 0.5% bupivacaine, or 0.75% ropivacaine.

FIGURE 4.35

a Femoral a.

b Adductor longus
m. tendon

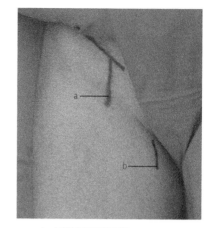

FIGURE 4.36

1 Obturator n. (anterior
branch)

2 Obturator n. (posterior
branch)

3 Adductor longus m.

4 Adductor brevis m.

5 Adductor magnus m.

6 Gracilis m.

7 Needle direction

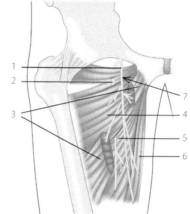

FIGURE 4.37 Direct
the needle cephalad and
dorsally.

a Needle insertion site

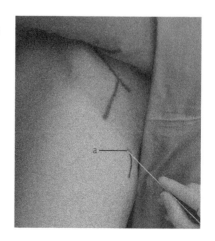

Obturator nerve block

COMPLEXITY: ⊗⊗⊗
See Figures 4.38 and 4.39.

Ultrasound-guided technique

Patient position: supine, with the leg to be blocked slightly externally rotated.

Landmarks: surface: adductor longus muscle; sonoanatomical: femur, adductor magnus, brevis and longus.

Technique: expose the groin and the medial aspect of the proximal thigh. Place a high-frequency linear transducer in the inguinal crease, and select a depth of field approximately 2–4 cm, although a greater depth may be required in obese patients. Obtain images in the SAX view, and scan slightly distally in the upper medial thigh. The obturator nerve in the upper thigh has divided into its posterior and anterior branches, lying above and below the adductor brevis. The branches of the obturator nerve are hyperechoic and may be accompanied by vessels.

Insert the needle perpendicular to the transducer and the ultrasound beam (OOP approach), and identify the anterior and posterior branches of the obturator nerve. Inject 5–10 mL of local anaesthetic in each of the two intermuscular fascial planes. Observe distension of the intermuscular planes and surrounding of the hyperechoic nerve structures by the local anaesthetic.

Needle: 22 G, 50 mm, insulated.

Local anaesthetic: 1% lignocaine, 0.5% bupivacaine, or 0.75% ropivacaine.

Comments: first, inject deep to the adductor brevis (posterior branch), then pull back and inject superficial to brevis (anterior branch).

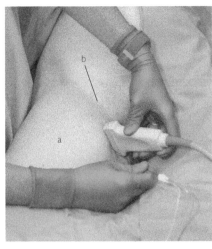

FIGURE 4.38 Insert the needle, using an OOP approach.

a   Right thigh
b   Right inguinal crease

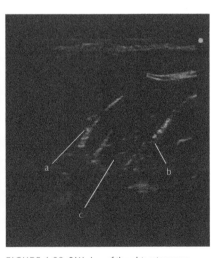

FIGURE 4.39 SAX view of the obturator nerve.

a   Anterior branch
b   Posterior branch
c   Adductor brevis

Sacral plexus block

COMPLEXITY: ✪✪✪

Indications
- Hip surgery
- Surgery of the sciatic distribution.

See Figures 4.40 and 4.41.

Technique

Patient position: lateral, with the leg to be anaesthetized superior and the hip flexed 60°.

Landmarks: PSIS and IT.

Technique: locate the PSIS, and draw a line connecting it to the IT. Insert the needle along this line, 40% from the PSIS, and advance along the sagittal plane. If bone is contacted, remove and redirect the needle 1–2 cm caudad and lateral to the previous insertion point. Brisk motor response of the ankle and foot at a stimulating current of 0.3 mA indicates correct needle placement. Inject 20 mL of anaesthetic slowly.

Needle: 22 G, 15 cm.

Local anaesthetic: 1.5% lignocaine with adrenaline 1:200 000 (30 mL), 0.5% bupivacaine, or 0.75% ropivacaine.

Comment: this technique uses similar landmarks to the psoas compartment (lumbar plexus) block and is useful for hip surgery when performed with the psoas compartment block. Isolated twitches of the hamstring muscles on stimulation also indicates correct needle placement. Twitching of the gluteus muscles indicates superficial needle placement. This is the easiest and most reliable landmark-based approach to the sciatic nerve.

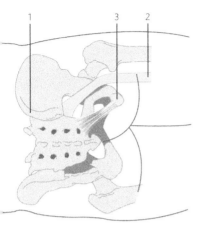

FIGURE 4.40

1   Posterior superior iliac spine
2   Sciatic n.
3   Ischial tuberosity

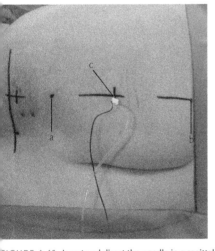

FIGURE 4.41 Insert and direct the needle in a sagittal plane.

a   Posterior superior iliac spine
b   Ischial tuberosity
c   Needle insertion site

Sciatic nerve block: subgluteal to popliteal fossa

COMPLEXITY: ✪✪✪

The sciatic nerve is a large structure and may be blocked at different levels to provide regional anaesthesia and analgesia for a wide range of indications. Consideration must be given to both the indication for the nerve block and the location where the sciatic nerve is best visualized with ultrasound to determine the best location to perform a block. Refer to Scanning tips for the lower extremities for a more detailed description of scanning the sciatic nerve.

Indications

- Hip surgery (proximal)
- Surgery of the sciatic distribution
- Leg surgery, when combined with a lumbar plexus block
- Analgesia (proximal for above the knee; distal for below the knee)
- Sympatholysis (achillodynia, diabetic gangrene, circulatory or wound-healing disorders, complex regional pain syndrome)
- Foot or ankle surgery.

See Figures 4.42 to 4.52.

Ultrasound-guided technique

Patient position: the patient may be positioned semi-prone, with the limb to be blocked uppermost (all approaches); supine, with the hip and knee flexed (distal sciatic block); or supine (anterior approach).

Landmarks: surface: superior iliac spine and ischial tuberosity, greater trochanter, and ischial tuberosity at gluteal fold and popliteal crease at knee; sonoanatomical: ischial tuberosity, greater trochanter, femur, and popliteal artery.

Technique: place a curved transducer (3–7 MHz) on the posterior thigh. The hyperechoic sciatic nerve may be identified between the gluteus maximus and adductor magnus muscles and posterior to the femur. In the mid-thigh, it may appear round or rectangular, while, distally, it appears circular and divides into two branches at its bifurcation. (Note: the nerve may be divided as proximal as the gluteal fold.) Distally, the sciatic nerve lies posterior (superficial) to the popliteal artery. Confirm nerve identity, and follow the course of the nerve by scanning proximally and distally to confirm anatomy before determining the appropriate level to block:

- Proximal sciatic (sacral plexus or subgluteal block) to block the hip
- Mid-thigh or more proximal sciatic to block the knee
- Distal sciatic, usually at or above the bifurcation, to block the knee and below.

An IP or OOP needle approach may be used; if using peripheral nerve stimulation, observe for an appropriately distal twitch. Inject 20–30 mL of local anaesthetic slowly to surround the nerve, observing spread.

Needle: 10–15 cm, stimulating for single shot; 10–15 cm, Tuohy for continuous blockade.

Local anaesthetic: 0.75% ropivacaine.

Comments: proximal (subgluteal) sciatic nerve may be difficult to identify with ultrasound, so landmarks may be required. Nerve stimulation is recommended if the nerve is deep.

FIGURE 4.42 Scan with a curvilinear probe to obtain a SAX view of the proximal sciatic nerve (patient in left lateral position).

a Greater trochanter

b Knee

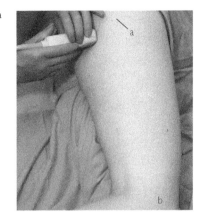

FIGURE 4.43 Scan with a linear probe to obtain a SAX view of the mid-femoral sciatic nerve; the needle is shown in an IP approach. The needle insertion point is on the groove between the biceps femoris and vastus lateralis muscles.

a Knee

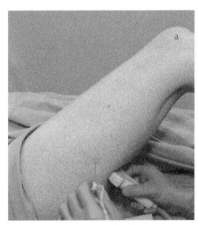

FIGURE 4.44 Scan with a linear probe to obtain a SAX view of the distal sciatic nerve.

a Knee

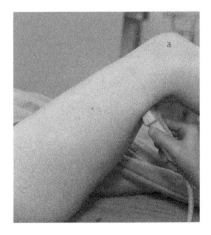

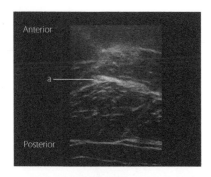

FIGURE 4.45 SAX view of the proximal sciatic nerve.

a   Sciatic n.

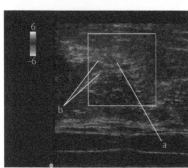

FIGURE 4.46 SAX view of the proximal sciatic nerve CFD.

a   Sciatic n.
b   Accompanying vessels

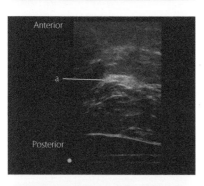

FIGURE 4.47 SAX view of the mid-femoral sciatic nerve.

a   Sciatic n.

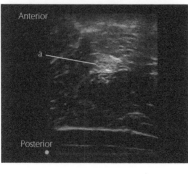

FIGURE 4.48 SAX view of the distal sciatic nerve.

a   Sciatic n.

FIGURE 4.49 SAX view of the sciatic nerve bifurcation.

a Common peroneal n.
b Tibial n.

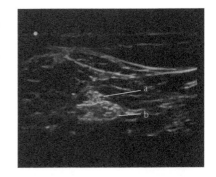

FIGURE 4.50 SAX view of the sciatic nerve bifurcation.

a Common peroneal n.
b Tibial n.

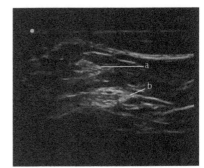

FIGURE 4.51 Probe position for proximal sciatic (subgluteal) block; insert the needle, using an IP approach.

a Greater trochanter
b Ischial tuberosity

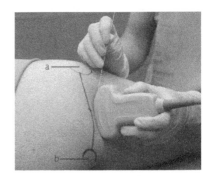

FIGURE 4.52 Probe position for distal sciatic (popliteal) block; insert the needle, using an IP approach.

a Femoral condyle
b Biceps femoris m. tendon

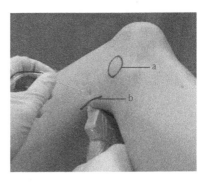

Sciatic nerve block: proximal anterior/ventral

COMPLEXITY: ⭐⭐⭐

Indications
- Leg surgery, when combined with lumbar plexus block
- Analgesia
- Sympathicolysis.

See Figures 4.53 to 4.56.

Ultrasound-guided technique

Patient position: supine.

Landmarks: surface: inguinal crease; sonoanatomical: femur, lesser trochanter, femoral artery.

Technique: place a curved, low-frequency (2–5 MHz) transducer on the thigh, approximately 8 cm from the inguinal crease. Ensure the needle trajectory is proximal to the femoral vessels entering the adductor canal. Observe the transverse view of the femur (short axis) as a curved hyperechoic line with an underlying bone shadow. Identify the lesser trochanter as the wide segment immediately above the femoral shaft by moving the transducer proximally and distally. The sciatic nerve may be identified in the proximal thigh, deep to the adductor muscles and posterior-medial to the femur, as predominantly hyperechoic and oval or elliptical in shape.

Visualization of the sciatic nerve may be improved by more medial orientation of the probe—anisotropy is an important determinant in optimizing sciatic sonoanatomy.

Both IP and OOP approaches may be used to perform this block. For the OOP approach, align the nerve target with the midpoint of the transducer and then insert the needle in the same location. Clear identification of the needle tip can be technically challenging when the needle angle is steep and the needle is deep inside the muscle layers. Walking the needle off the medial aspect of the femoral shaft may assist with needle placement. Confirm needle-to-nerve contact by electrical stimulation, and observe local anaesthetic spread, or by jiggling the needle. Alternatively, hydrodissection may be performed, using 5% dextrose to maintain electrical stimulation.

The IP approach is more difficult to perform, as the contralateral leg often obstructs the needle trajectory. Insert the needle on the medial side of the ultrasound transducer, following infiltration of the skin with local anaesthetic. Advance the needle in a medial to lateral direction, in addition to an anterior to posterior direction, medial to the femoral neurovascular bundle (displaced laterally once the thigh is externally rotated). The steep angle of needle advancement may make it difficult to clearly visualize the block needle. Nerve movement may indicate contact with the needle. It is recommended that electrical stimulation be used for additional confirmation. Inject 20–30 mL of local anaesthetic around the sciatic nerve for post-operative analgesia.

Needle: 20 G, 15 cm, insulated block.

Local anaesthetic: 0.75% ropivacaine.

Comments: a single injection site may be sufficient, with adequate local anaesthesia spread around the nerve. Failing this, the needle may be withdrawn slightly and repositioned so that local anaesthetic is deposited on the medial and lateral aspects of the nerve. This block is very well tolerated by patients if performed following femoral nerve block for knee surgery.

FIGURE 4.53 Use a curvilinear probe, and insert the needle, using an OOP approach.

a Right thigh
b Abdomen

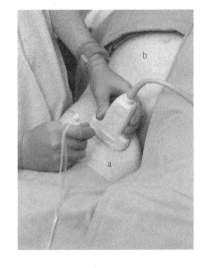

FIGURE 4.54 Close-up SAX view of the anterior sciatic.

a Femoral vessels and n.
b Femur
c Sciatic n.

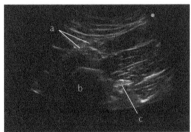

FIGURE 4.55 SAX deep view of the anterior sciatic.

a Femoral n. and vessels
b Femur
c Sciatic n.

FIGURE 4.56 SAX view of the anterior sciatic CFD.

a Femoral a. and femoral v. (and femoral n.)
b Femur
c Sciatic n.

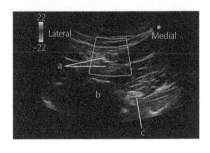

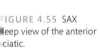

Saphenous nerve block

COMPLEXITY: ⬤⬤⬡

Ultrasound guidance may facilitate the success of saphenous nerve blocks, as the success rate for traditional landmark techniques is only 33%.

Indications

- Anaesthesia supplementary to incomplete lumbar plexus block (medial lower leg)
- Complete anaesthesia of the lower leg, in combination with a sciatic nerve block.

See Figures 4.57 to 4.60.

Ultrasound-guided technique

Patient position: supine, with the leg externally rotated and hip and knee flexed.

Landmarks: sonoanatomical: femoral nerve, artery and vein, sartorius muscle.

Technique: place a high-frequency, linear-array ultrasound probe on the mid-thigh over the sartorius muscle, which runs lateral to medial from the ASIS to the tibia across the anterior thigh. In the SAX view, observe the sartorius muscle overlying the femoral vessels proximal to the adductor canal. The terminal branches of the femoral nerve, of which the saphenous nerve is the major branch, lie adjacent to the femoral artery. Alternatively, if this view is difficult to obtain, commence scanning in the inguinal region for the femoral vessels in a SAX orientation. Trace down the femoral artery distally until the sartorius muscle forms a roof over the artery and saphenous nerve, proximal to the adductor canal.

Perform the block, using an OOP or IP approach, ensuring local anaesthetic deposition is below the saphenous muscle, and hydrodissect around the nerves surrounding the femoral artery.

Needle: 25 G, 6 cm.

Local anaesthetic: 1% ropivacaine.

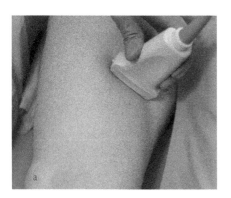

FIGURE 4.57   Probe position for SAX view of the saphenous nerve.

a   Right knee

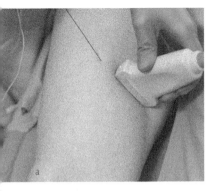

FIGURE 4.58 Needle insertion, using an IP approach.

a Right knee

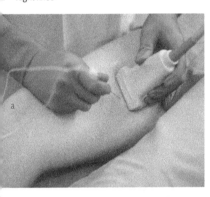

FIGURE 4.59 Needle insertion, using an OOP approach.

a Right knee

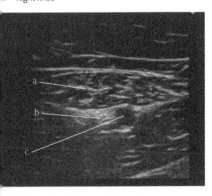

FIGURE 4.60 SAX view of the saphenous n.

a Sartorius m.

b Saphenous n.

c Femoral a.

Ankle blocks

COMPLEXITY: ●●●

The foot is supplied by five nerves: four originate in the sciatic nerve (superficial and deep peroneal nerves, tibial and sural nerves), and the other (saphenous nerve) is the terminal branch of the femoral nerve. This block is often painful to perform, and the patient may require sedation to tolerate its placement.

Indications

- Anaesthesia supplementary to incomplete lumbosacral plexus block
- Foot surgery
- Analgesia
- Diagnostic block.

See Figures 4.61, 4.62, and 4.63.

Technique

Superficial peroneal nerve

Supplies the skin on the back of the foot and toes, except an area between the great and second toes.

Patient position: supine.

Landmarks: tibia (anterior edge) and lateral malleolus (upper edge).

Technique: insert the needle between the anterior edge of the tibia and the upper edge of the lateral malleolus, approximately a hand-width above the lateral malleolus. Infiltrate the area subcutaneously with 5–10 mL of anaesthetic.

Sural nerve

Supplies the lateral edge of the foot and is variable up to the fifth toe.

Patient position: supine.

Landmarks: Achilles tendon and lateral malleolus.

Technique: insert the needle between the Achilles tendon and the lateral malleolus, approximately a hand-width above the lateral malleolus. Infiltrate the area subcutaneously with 5 mL of anaesthetic.

Saphenous nerve

Supplies the skin medially from the inner ankle and is variable up to the great toe.

Patient position: supine.

Landmarks: tibia (anterior edge) and medial malleolus.

Technique: insert the needle at the anterior edge of the tibia, approximately a hand-width above the medial malleolus. Infiltrate the area subcutaneously with 5–10 mL of anaesthetic, from the anterior edge of the tibia to the Achilles tendon.

Needle: 22–24 G, 4–6 cm.

Local anaesthetic: 1% lignocaine, 0.5% bupivacaine, or 0.75% ropivacaine.

Comments: if these subcutaneous blocks are initially performed as a ring infiltration, subsequent needle-sticks will be pain-free.

FIGURE 4.61

a Extensor digitorum longus m. tendon
b Dorsalis pedis a.
c Medial malleolus
d Lateral malleolus

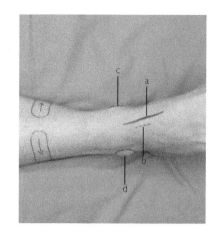

FIGURE 4.62

1 Sural n.
2 Superficial peroneal n.
3 Deep peroneal n.

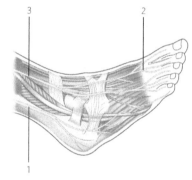

FIGURE 4.63
Subcutaneous ring infiltration above the ankle to block the superficial peroneal and sural nerves (lateral) and saphenous nerve (medial).

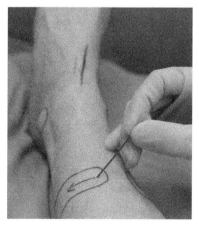

Ankle blocks

COMPLEXITY: ●●●
See Figures 4.64 to 4.67.

Technique

Deep peroneal nerve

Supplies the medial side of the great toe and the lateral side of the second toe.

Patient position: supine.

Landmarks: extensor digitorum longus muscle (tendon) and dorsalis pedis artery.

Technique: palpate the tendon of the extensor digitorum longus muscle. Insert the needle between the tendon and the dorsalis pedis artery, perpendicular to the skin. Advance the needle slightly under the artery. Inject 2–5 mL of anaesthetic, following negative aspiration.

Needle: 24 G, 3–5 cm.

Local anaesthetic: 1% lignocaine, 0.5% bupivacaine, or 0.75% ropivacaine (2–3 mL).

Posterior tibial nerve

Supplies the sole of the feet, with the exception of the extreme lateral and proximal segments.

Patient position: supine, with the leg of the foot to be blocked rotated externally.

Landmarks: posterior tibial artery, Achilles tendon, and medial malleolus.

Technique: insert the needle directly dorsal to the posterior tibial artery on the medial side of the joint or, alternatively, directly anterior of the Achilles tendon at the level of the medial malleolus. Insert the needle perpendicular to the skin. Inject 3–8 mL of anaesthetic while aspirating intermittently.

Needle: 22 or 24 G, 5 cm, insulated.

Local anaesthetic: 1% lignocaine, 0.5% bupivacaine, or 0.75% ropivacaine (3–4 mL).

Comments: nerve stimulation is recommended. Plantarflexion of the toes indicates correct needle placement.

FIGURE 4.64

1 Superficial peroneal n.
2 Saphenous n.
3 Dorsalis pedis a.
4 Deep peroneal n.

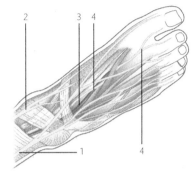

FIGURE 4.65 Insert the needle perpendicular to the skin.

a Extensor digitorum longus m. tendon
b Dorsalis pedis a.
c Needle insertion site

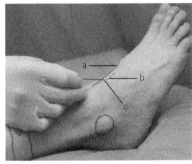

FIGURE 4.66

1 Saphenous n.
2 Posterior tibial a.
3 Tibial n.

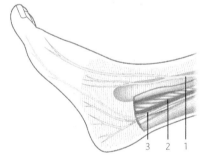

FIGURE 4.67 Insert the needle dorsal of the artery and perpendicular to the skin.

a Posterior tibial a.
b Medial malleolus
c Needle insertion site

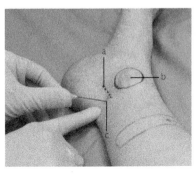

Ankle blocks

COMPLEXITY: ⬤⬤⬤
See Figures 4.68 to 4.71.

Ultrasound-guided technique

As the superficial peroneal, saphenous, and sural nerves can be blocked by subcutaneous infiltration, ultrasound guidance is only recommended for blocks of the deep peroneal and posterior tibial nerves. Prior to blocking the deep peroneal or posterior tibial nerve, block the superficial peroneal, sural, and saphenous nerves by subcutaneous infiltration (as described in the previous sections) with 5–8 mL of anaesthetic.

Deep peroneal nerve

Patient position: supine.

Landmarks: surface: tibia (anterior edge); sonoanatomical: anterior tibial and dorsalis pedis arteries.

Technique: place a linear ultrasound probe lateral to the anterior edge of the tibia, about 5 cm proximal to the foot. Locate the anterior tibial artery, which continues as the dorsalis pedis artery in the foot. Colour flow Doppler and the pulsatile nature of the artery will confirm the location of the artery. Lateral to the artery, the hyperechoic deep peroneal nerve is visualized. Using an OOP approach, deposit 3–4 mL of anaesthetic around the nerve after confirming needle placement with a test dose of anaesthetic.

Needle: 22 G, Stimuplex®.

Local anaesthetic: 0.75% ropivacaine or 1:1 mixture of 1% lignocaine and 0.75% ropivacaine.

Posterior tibial nerve

Patient position: supine, with the hip and knee flexed and the foot placed across the contralateral leg to expose the medial malleolus.

Landmarks: surface: medial malleolus; sonoanatomical: posterior tibial artery.

Technique: place the linear-array probe 5 cm above the medial malleolus, and locate the posterior tibial artery. Confirm this either by its pulsatile nature or with colour flow Doppler. The tibial nerve is the hyperechoic structure posterior to the artery. Using an OOP approach, inject 3–4 mL of anaesthetic slowly after confirming needle placement with a test dose of anaesthetic.

Needle: 22 G, Stimuplex®.

Local anaesthetic: 0.75% ropivacaine or 1:1 mixture of 1% lignocaine and 0.75% ropivacaine.

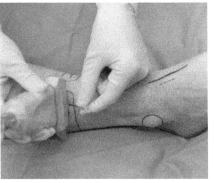

FIGURE 4.68
Insert the needle lateral to the anterior tibial artery, using an OOP approach.

FIGURE 4.69 SAX
view of the deep
peroneal nerve.

a   Anterior tibial a.
b   Deep peroneal n.
c   Tibia

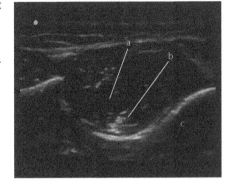

FIGURE 4.70 Insert
the needle, using an
OOP approach.

a   Medial malleolus

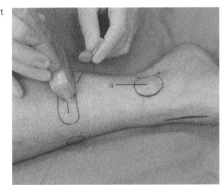

FIGURE 4.71 SAX
view of the posterior
tibial nerve.

a   Posterior tibial a.
b   Posterior tibial n.

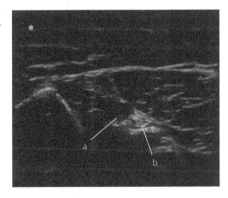

References

1 Perlas A and Chan V. Ultrasound-assisted nerve blocks. New York: New York School of Regional Anaesthesia. Viewed 19 October 2009, <http://www.nysora.com/peripheral_nerve_blocks/ultrasound-guided_techniques/3063-ultrasound_assisted_nerve_blocks.html>.

2 Winnie A, Ramamurthy S, Durrnai Z (1973). The inguinal paravascular technic of lumbar plexus anesthesia: the '3-in-1 block'. *Anesth Analg* **52**, 989–96.

3 Ganapathy S, Wassserman R, Watson J, *et al.* (1999). Modified continuous femoral three-in-one block for postoperative pain after total knee arthroplasty. *Anesth Analg* **89**, 1197–202.

4 Dalens B, Vanneuville G, Tanguy A (1989). Comparison of the fascia iliaca compartment block with the 3-in-1 block in children. *Anesth Analg* **69**, 705–13.

CHAPTER FIVE

SPINE AND PARA-AXIAL REGION

Anatomy of the spine and para-axial region

See Figure 5.1.

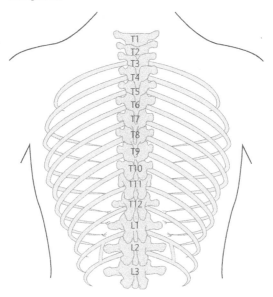

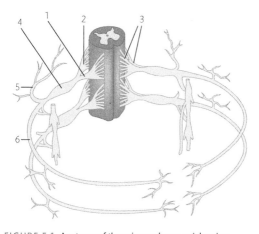

FIGURE 5.1 Anatomy of the spine and para-axial region.

1	Ventral root	4	Dorsal ramus ganglion
2	Dorsal root	5	Dorsal ramus
3	Rootlets	6	Ventral ramus (intercostal)

Sensory supply

See Figure 5.2.

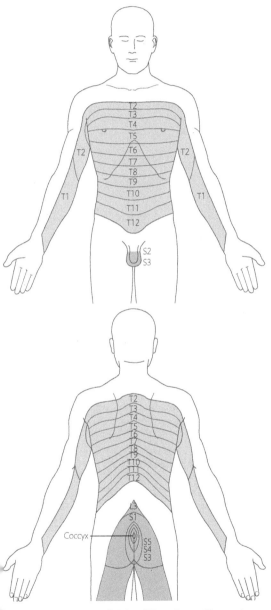

FIGURE 5.2 Sensory supply. T1 and T2 send nerve fibres to the upper limbs and the upper thorax; T3–T6 supply the thorax; T7–T11 supply the lower thorax and abdomen, and T12 innervates the abdominal wall and the skin of the front part of the gluteal region.

Thoracic paravertebral block

COMPLEXITY: ✪✪✪

Indications
• Breast and axillary surgery
• Pain management after thoracic surgery or rib fractures.

Side effects and complications
• Total spinal anaesthesia
• Epidural anaesthesia
• Quadratus femoris muscle weakness can occur when the spinous process levels are not determined accurately and the levels below L1 are blocked.

See Figures 5.3, 5.4, and 5.5.

Technique

Patient position: sitting or lateral decubitus and kyphotic. If sitting, rest the patient's feet on a stool to increase comfort and the degree of kyphosis.

Landmarks: midline of spinous processes (relevant to the anaesthesia).

Technique: locate the midline of, and outline, each spinous process. After subcutaneous infiltration, insert the needle perpendicular to the skin, 2.5 cm lateral from the midline at the level of the spinous process requiring anaesthesia. Advance the needle towards to the transverse process. After contacting the transverse process, note the needle depth; withdraw the needle to the skin; redirect 10° cephalad, and re-advance. 'Step off' the transverse process, and advance the needle 1–1.5 cm further, using a loss-of-resistance technique with saline (a subtle loss of resistance is felt). If difficulty is experienced with locating space, redirect the needle 10° caudad and re-advance. Inject 4–5 mL of anaesthetic into the paravertebral space. Repeat for each spinous process requiring anaesthesia. The cephalad-caudad space between the first two transverse processes anaesthetized can be used to locate the remaining transverse processes requiring anaesthesia. For breast surgery, a single injection of 20 mL only at T3 or T4 is required. Placement of this dose via catheter is recommended.

Needle: 18 G, 8 cm, Tuohy.

Local anaesthetic: 2% lignocaine with adrenaline 1:200 000, 0.5% bupivacaine with adrenaline 1:200 000, or 0.5% ropivacaine.

Comments: ultrasound is useful to locate the position and depth of the transverse process. Kyphosis increases the distance between adjacent transverse processes and assists needle progression beyond the transverse process. Patients may experience moderate discomfort and may require sedation. Directing the needle medially will increase the risk of epidural or spinal injection and laterally will increase the risk of pneumothorax. The depth at which the needle contacts the transverse process varies, according to the patient's habitus and the level of the spinous process. In the average patient, contact with the transverse process at T1 and T2, and L4 and L5 occurs at 6–8 cm needle depth, whereas, at T5 and T10, contact occurs at 2–4 cm needle depth. Recent evidence suggests this block reduces phantom pain post-mastectomy and may reduce breast cancer recurrence.[1]

FIGURE 5.3
a Midline of the
   spinous processes
b Paramedial line
   2.5 cm lateral to the
   midline
c Needle insertion site

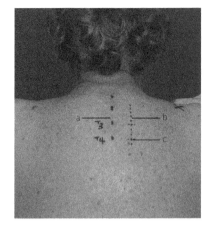

FIGURE 5.4
1 Spinal n.
2 Transverse process
3 Spinous process

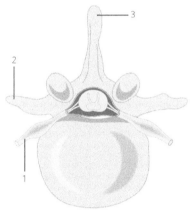

FIGURE 5.5 Insert
and advance the needle
in a sagittal direction.

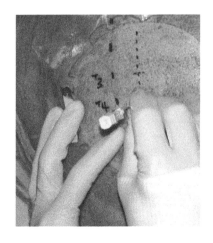

Thoracic paravertebral block

COMPLEXITY: ✪✪✪
See Figures 5.6, 5.7, and 5.8.

Continuous catheter technique

Technique: locate the paravertebral space, as described. Inject an initial bolus of 5 mL of anaesthetic into the paravertebral space. Advance the catheter 3–5 cm beyond the needle tip; if the catheter does not feed easily, repeat the block. Secure the catheter to the skin with clear dressing, and complete the block via catheter. Infuse the anaesthetic at a rate of 10 mL/hour, or 6 mL/hour if a patient-controlled analgesia is planned.

Equipment: 18 G, Tuohy needle and catheter.

Local anaesthetic: initial bolus: 0.5% bupivacaine or 0.5% ropivacaine; continuous infusion: 0.25% bupivacaine or 0.2% ropivacaine.

Comments: to manage breakthrough pain, administer a bolus of anaesthetic through the catheter; increasing the rate of infusion is rarely adequate. If pain is unrelieved after 30 minutes, the catheter should be considered dislodged and removed.

FIGURE 5.6 (a) Insert the needle, and contact the transverse process of the individual vertebrae (note the depth of contact, usually 2–4 cm). (b) Withdraw the needle to the skin, and re-advance cephalad at a 10° angle. 'Step off' the transverse process, and advance 1 cm deeper.

1   Spinous processes
2   Transverse processes
3   Spinal nerves

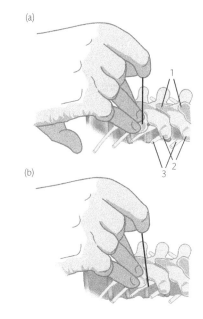

(a)

(b)

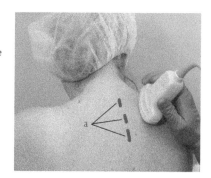

FIGURE 5.7 Scanning with a curvilinear probe is useful to locate the position and depth of the transverse processes.

a   Thoracic spine

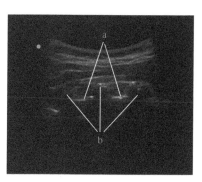

FIGURE 5.8 Thoracic paravertebral block.

a   Paravertebral space
b   Transverse process.

Epidural block for labour anaesthesia

COMPLEXITY: ✪✪✪

Indications
• Anaesthesia and analgesia during labour.

Specific contraindications
• Recent antepartum haemorrhage
• Cephalopelvic disproportion.

Side effects and complications
• Accidental puncture of the dura
• Haematoma, owing to puncture of an epidural vein
• Intravascular or intrathecal injection
• Total spinal block, owing to intrathecal injection
• Uterine hypotension (when higher concentrations of anaesthetic are injected, e.g. 0.25% bupivacaine)
• Post-dural puncture headache
• Meningitis.
See Figures 5.9, 5.10, and 5.11.

Continuous catheter technique (midline approach)

Patient position: left lateral or sitting.

Landmarks: iliac crest and midline of L2–L4 spinous processes.

Technique: palpate and draw a line between the iliac crests to estimate the level of the L3–L4 spinous processes. Raise a subcutaneous bleb of anaesthetic between two adjacent vertebrae (L2–L3 or L3–L4), and infiltrate deeper in the midline and paraspinously to anaesthetize the needle insertion site and posterior structures. Insert the epidural needle sagittally between two adjacent vertebrae. Direct and advance the needle slightly cephalad and slowly through the supraspinous ligament and the interspinous ligament (2–3 cm). When the needle is advanced into the ligamentum flavum, increased resistance is usually felt. Control the needle's movement by gripping its wing and resting the dorsum of the non-injecting hand against the patient's back. Attach a loss-of-resistance syringe with 5–8 mL of air or a syringe with saline. With continuous pressure on the syringe plunger, advance the needle slowly until its tip exits the ligamentum flavum and enters the epidural space. A loss of resistance or 'click' (rare) may be felt. Advance the epidural catheter 4–6 cm past the needle tip (never withdraw the catheter through the needle—this risks shearing the catheter), and inject a 5–10 mL bolus of anaesthetic through the catheter. Inject the bolus in 5 mL increments, aspirating carefully between increments and checking the level to ensure the catheter is not subarachnoid. The addition of adrenaline (1:200 000) may reveal intravascular catheter placement if tachycardia is induced. Fix the catheter, and infuse anaesthetic at a rate of 5–10 mL/hour.

Equipment: 16 or 18 G, 8 cm Tuohy needle and 18 or 20 G catheter.

Local anaesthetic: initial bolus: 0.125–0.5% bupivacaine or 0.2–0.5% ropivacaine; continuous infusion: 0.125% bupivacaine or 0.2% ropivacaine.

Comment: as the interspinous ligament is extremely dense, injection into it is almost impossible. It is not necessary to anaesthetize above the level of the L1–L2 spinous processes for labour analgesia, and it has the increased risk of spinal cord injury. The addition of 2 micrograms/mL of fentanyl produces a better-quality block and reduces anaesthetic requirements.

FIGURE 5.9

a L3–L5 spinous processes

b Needle insertion site

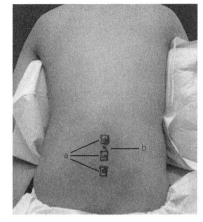

FIGURE 5.10

1 Spinous process

2 Spinal cord within dura

3 Nerve root

4 Vertebral body

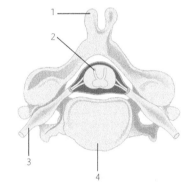

FIGURE 5.11 Direct the needle in a sagittal plane.

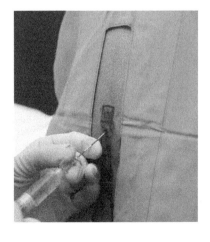

Intercostal block

COMPLEXITY: ⊗⊗⊗

Indications
• Analgesia for chest trauma, such as rib fractures
• Analgesia following surgery of the chest and upper abdominal area, such as thoracotomy, thoracostomy, mastectomy, gastrostomy, and cholecystectomy.

Specific contraindications
• Haemostatic deficiencies
• When pneumothorax would be fatal.

Side effects and complications
• Pneumothorax and lung injury
• Toxicity is a concern, owing to the rapid absorption of anaesthetic from the intercostal space.
See Figures 5.12 and 5.13.

Technique
Patient position: prone, sitting, or lateral, with block side up. If the patient is prone, place a pillow under their abdomen, with their arms hanging to the side. Patients who are sitting should lean forward, holding a pillow, and be supported with their arms forward. The scapulae pull laterally in both positions, facilitating access to the posterior rib angles above T7.

Landmarks: rib (inferior edge) and erector spinae muscles.

Technique: of the ribs to be anesthetized, mark their inferior edges just lateral to the erector spinae muscle group (usually 6–8 cm and 4–7 cm from the midline of the lower and upper ribs, respectively). Infiltrate the area subcutaneously. Palpate the needle insertion site, and draw the skin approximately 1 cm cephalad. Insert the needle cephalad (bevel facing cephalad) at a 20° angle. Advance the needle until it contacts the rib (less than 1 cm for most non-obese patients). A small volume of anaesthetic may be injected to anaesthetize the periosteum. Gently 'step' the needle caudad, and allow the skin to move back over the rib. Advance the needle 3 mm further, maintaining the 20° cephalad angle. Aspirate for blood, and then inject 5–10 mL per rib anaesthetic. Repeat for all ribs that require anaesthesia.

Needle: 22 or 24 G, 4–5 cm.

Local anaesthetic: 1% lignocaine with adrenaline 1:200 000, 0.5% bupivacaine, or 0.75% ropivacaine.

Comments: for a single intercostal nerve block, it is desirable to block one intercostal nerve cephalad and one caudad. To ensure the needle tip remains fixed and unaffected by hand and chest movement, connect the needle to the syringe with extension tubing, and have an assistant perform the aspiration and injection.

FIGURE 5.12

1 Interpleural space
2 Subserous fascia
3 Endothoracic fascia
4 Intercostal v.
5 Intercostal a.
6 intercostal n.
7 Internal intercostal m.

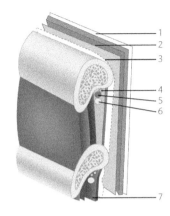

FIGURE 5.13 Direct
the needle cephalad at a
20° angle.

a Rib (inferior edge)
b Spinous processes
c Needle insertion site

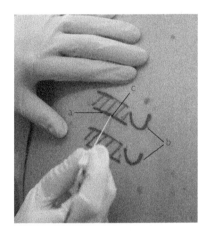

Intercostal block

Ultrasound-guided technique

Patient position: sitting, with patient leaning forward, holding a pillow, and supported with their arms forward. The scapulae pull laterally, facilitating access to the posterior rib angles above T7.

Landmarks: surface: midline of spinous processes; sonoanatomical: inner and intermediate intercostalis muscles, and parietal pleura.

Technique: place the linear-array ultrasound probe longitudinally 5 cm from the midline of the spinous processes. Locate the intercostal space of interest, seen between the two ribs as bony landmarks. Rotate the probe into a transverse view along the intercostal space, imaging the inner and intermediate intercostal muscles, parietal pleura, and neurovascular bundle under the rib. Colour flow Doppler, or the pulsatile nature on 2D echo, will identify the intercostal artery. Using an IP approach, insert the needle on the medial aspect of the probe, and advance the needle tip to above the parietal pleura and intercostal muscles adjacent to the intercostal artery. Confirm needle placement with a test dose of anaesthetic, and aspirate for blood. Inject 5–7 mL of anaesthetic per rib. Repeat for all ribs that require anaesthesia.

Needle: 25 G, 5 cm.

Local anaesthetic: 0.75% ropivacaine or 1:1 mixture of 1% lignocaine and 0.75% ropivacaine.

Comments: ultrasound-guided intercostal nerve block provides a distinct advantage over the traditional technique, as pain and swelling of overlying tissue may prevent rib palpation in some patients. Ultrasound also allows for rapid screening of post-procedure pneumothorax.

FIGURE 5.14 Place the probe longitudinally 5 cm from the midline of the spinous processes.

a   Spinous processes

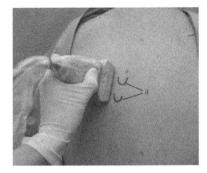

FIGURE 5.15 Longitudinal SAX view of the intercostal space.

a   Rib (with dorsal shadowing)
b   Intercostal mm.
c   Neurovascular bundle
d   Parietal pleura

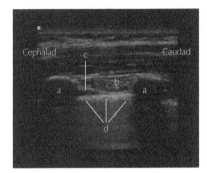

FIGURE 5.16 Rotate the probe into a transverse view along the intercostal space, and insert the needle using an IP approach (medial aspect of probe).

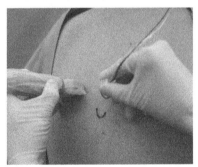

FIGURE 5.17 Transverse oblique SAX view of the intercostal space.

a   Rib (with dorsal shadowing)
b   Neurovascular bundle
c   Parietal pleura

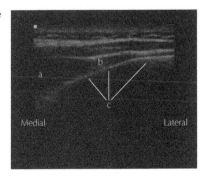

Posterior transversus abdominis plane (TAP) block

COMPLEXITY: ⚫⚫⚫

Nine segments from the anterior rami of the T6–L1 spinal nerves innervate the abdominal wall. These nerves pass inferoanteriorly from the intercostal spaces and run in a neurovascular plane between the internal oblique and transversus abdominis muscles. This is known as the transversus abdominis plane (TAP). The lateral branch arises from the mid-axillary line and innervates the abdominal wall to the edge of the rectus abdominis muscle. The anterior branch passes forward in the TAP to penetrate the muscle layers and supply afferents to the anterior abdominal wall.

Thoracoabdominal nerves arising from T7–T9 innervate the skin superior to the umbilicus, those arising from T10 innervate the skin around the umbilicus, and those arising from T11, T12 (cutaneous branches of the subcostal nerve), and L1 (iliohypogastric and ilioinguinal nerves) innervate the skin inferior to the umbilicus.

Indications

- Anaesthesia and analgesia of the somatic abdominal wall from the pubis to the level of the umbilicus without neuraxial blockade
- Abdominal wall operations (laparotomy, appendicectomy, hernia repairs, Caesarean section, and hysterectomy).

See Figures 5.18, 5.19, and 5.20.

Ultrasound-guided technique

Patient position: supine.

Landmarks: surface: lateral abdominal wall, umbilicus, iliac crest, lower costal margin; sonoanatomical: external and internal oblique, and transversus abdominis muscles.

Technique: place a high-frequency ultrasound probe on the anterior abdominal wall, on an angle along the line connecting the ASIS to the subcostal margin, midway between the iliac crest and the ribs. Insert the needle, using an IP approach, directed medial to lateral, in position between the transversus abdominis and internal oblique muscles. Local anaesthetic should be deposited deep to the fascial layer that separates these muscles. Aim to concentrate the local anaesthesia between the ASIS and the anterior axillary line to block T10–L1. Confirm needle placement with a test dose of anaesthetic or saline. Following negative aspiration, inject 20 mL of anaesthetic slowly in divided boluses, advancing the needle within the hydrodissected space to open the TAP. The anaesthetic solution should spread widely, forming a hypoechoic 'lens' within the TAP as it hydrodissects the plane between the internal oblique and the transversus abdominis muscles. Repeat on the opposite side for a bilateral block. If the plane is unclear, choose to inject between the transversus muscle and its more superficial fascia.

Needle: 21 or 22 G, 8–12 cm.

Local anaesthetic: 0.2–0.5% ropivacaine.

Comments: unless the procedure is for surgery within the anterior abdominal wall, TAP block must be administered in conjunction with multimodal analgesia for visceral or pelvic components of surgery. The amount of anaesthetic and opioids administered may be reduced. This description differs slightly from the classical approach and minimizes sparing of the L1 dermatome.

FIGURE 5.18

1. Branch of the anterior cutaneous n.
2. Rectus abdominis m.
3. External oblique m.
4. Internal oblique m.
5. Branch of the lateral cutaneous n.
6. Transversus abdominis m.

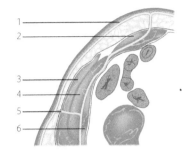

FIGURE 5.19

Insert the needle, using an IP approach, directed medial to lateral.

a. Costal margin

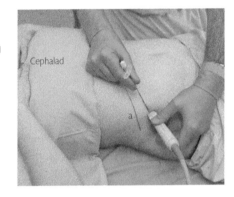

FIGURE 5.20

Posterior TAP block.

a. Adipose tissue
b. External oblique m.
c. Internal oblique m.
d. TAP
e. Transversus abdominis m.
f. Peritoneal contents

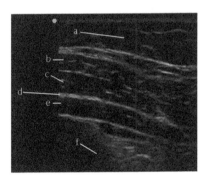

Subcostal TAP block

COMPLEXITY: ★★★
The posterior TAP block does not reliably produce analgesia above the umbilicus. The subcostal TAP block is a modification of the original technique, created to extend the analgesia provided by the posterior TAP block above the umbilicus.[2]

Indications
• Laparotomy incisions extending above the umbilicus.
See Figures 5.21 to 5.24.

Ultrasound-guided technique
Patient position: supine.

Landmarks: surface: costal margin, xiphoid process;
sonoanatomical: transversus abdominis plane.

Technique: place a high-frequency ultrasound probe perpendicular to the abdominal wall, just beneath and parallel to the costal margin, but oblique to the sagittal plane. Adjust the field depth to 2–6 cm. Introduce the needle, using an IP approach, near the xiphoid process, starting from medial to lateral along the subcostal trajectory. Initial deposition of local anaesthetic is between the transversus abdominis and the rectus abdominis muscles, or between the rectus and the posterior rectus sheath if the transversus is not behind the rectus at that level. Injection of 1–2 mL of local anaesthetic opens the insertion plane between the rectus and transversus, allowing advancement of the needle into the space hydrodissected by the local anaesthetic. Hydrodissection is used to open the transversus plane progressively; the needle is intermittently advanced, parallel to the costal margin and towards the iliac crest, with subsequent small injections of local anaesthetic. Ensure the needle stays within the transversus plane and does not pass superficial to the internal oblique at the lateral rectus edge. This technique lends itself well as a continuous catheter technique; a catheter may be placed down the needle which then lies largely along the transversus plane, with the tip near the iliac crest. Local anaesthetic infused down the catheter passes back up the transversus plane that was previously opened by hydrodissection.

Needle: 10–15 cm, Tuohy, or 22 G, 10–15 cm.

Local anaesthetic: 0.2–0.375% ropivacaine, 30 mL volume each side.

FIGURE 5.21 Insert
the needle, using an
IP approach, directed
medial to lateral.

a Costal margin

b ASIS

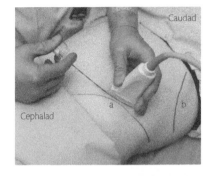

FIGURE 5.22
Subcostal TAP.

a Rectus

b Peritoneal contents

c External oblique m.

d Internal oblique m.

e TAP

f Transversus
abdominis m.

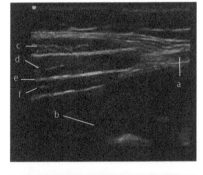

FIGURE 5.23
Subcostal
TAP—correct plane.

a Local anaesthetic in
internal oblique plane
(incorrect placement)

b Tuohy needle

c Local anaesthetic
hydrodissection in TAP

d External oblique m.

e Internal oblique m.

f Transversus
abdominis m.

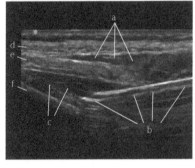

FIGURE 5.24
Subcostal TAP catheter.

a Local anaesthetic

b Bevel of Tuohy needle

c Catheter entering
hydrodissected TAP

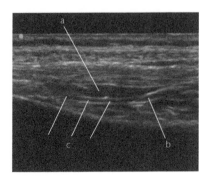

Rectus sheath block

The anterior divisions of spinal segmental nerves that innervate the abdominal wall run laterally between the transverse abdominis and internal oblique muscle layers. These nerves then enter the lateral edge of the rectus sheath and run posterior to the rectus muscle on the sheath. The nerves then variably pierce the muscle and travel anteriorly to innervate the medial anterior abdominal wall. Injection of local anaesthetic into the plane between the posterior rectus sheath and the posterior rectus muscle may be used to block these nerves.

Indications

- Epigastric hernia repair, in combination with light general anaesthesia
- Post-operative analgesia following midline laparotomy.

See Figures 5.25 to 5.28.

Ultrasound-guided technique

Patient position: supine.

Landmarks: surface: umbilicus; sonoanatomical: rectus abdominis muscle.

Technique: place a high-frequency ultrasound probe in an axial (transverse) plane at the level of the umbilicus; scan laterally, and identify the lateral edge of the rectus muscle. Visualize the three layers of the rectus sheath corresponding to linea semilunaris. Introduce the needle, using an IP approach. Identify the lateral edge of the rectus muscle, and place the needle deep to the muscle and superficial to the posterior rectus sheath at this point. Correct needle placement may be confirmed by first injecting saline and using ultrasound to observe the spread of injectate between the rectus muscle and posterior sheath. Inject 5–10 mL of local anaesthetic. Depending on the size and location of the surgical incision, three or four injection sites, approximately 5 cm apart, may be used bilaterally.

Needle: 21 or 22 G.

Local anaesthetic: 0.25–0.75% ropivacaine, 5–10 mL for each point up to a total 40 mL volume.

FIGURE 5.25 Insert the needle, using an IP approach, lateral to the umbilicus.

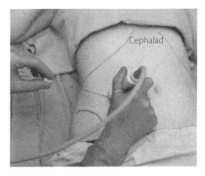

FIGURE 5.26 Linea alba.

a   Linea alba

b   Rectus mm.

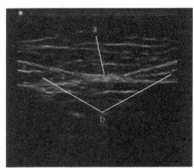

FIGURE 5.27 Rectus muscle.

a   Rectus

b   External oblique m.

c   Internal oblique m.

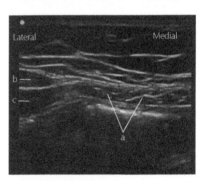

FIGURE 5.28 Rectus lateral border.

a   Linea semilunaris

b   Rectus m.

c   End point of needle in IP approach

d   External oblique m.

e   Internal oblique m.

f   Transversus abdominis m.

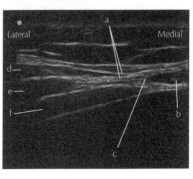

Ilioinguinal iliohypogastric block

Indications
• Analgesia following inguinal hernia repair.
See Figures 5.29 and 5.30.

Ultrasound-guided technique
Patient position: supine.

Landmarks: surface: iliac crest, umbilicus; sonoanatomical: anterior superior iliac spine (ASIS).

Technique: place a linear 10–15 MHz transducer obliquely along a line joining the ASIS and the umbilicus, immediately superior and medial to the ASIS. The three muscular layers of the abdominal wall are identified: the external oblique, the internal oblique, and the transverse abdominis muscles. It is expected the ilioinguinal and iliohypogastric nerves—often hyperechoic in appearance—will lie between the transverse abdominis and internal oblique muscles above the ASIS. Small vessels will commonly be visualized adjacent to both nerves within the same plane. Colour Doppler may be used to confirm vascular identity.

Insert the needle parallel to, and in line with, the transducer and ultrasound beam (IP approach), visualizing the needle shaft and tip during advancement. Accuracy of needle position may be confirmed by injecting test boluses of local anaesthetic or normal saline. Inaccurate placement of the needle within a muscle layer will result in the visualization of intramuscular fluid injection. Correct placement of the needle is indicated by fluid expansion in the space bounded by the hyperechoic fascial sheath of the internal oblique and transverse abdominis muscle layers; inject 10–15 mL of local anaesthetic into this plane.

Needle: 22 G, 5–8 cm.

Local anaesthetic: 0.2–0.75% ropivacaine.

Comments: the same volume of local anaesthetic may be deposited around the vessels in the fascial plane if the ilioinguinal or iliohypogastric nerves are not visualized.

FIGURE 5.29 Insert the needle, using an IP approach.

a Costal margin
b ASIS

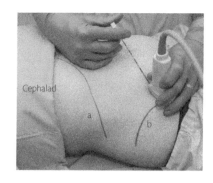

FIGURE 5.30 SAX view of the ilioinguinal iliohypogastric nerve.

a Blood vessel
b ASIS
c Ilioinguinal iliohypogastric n.

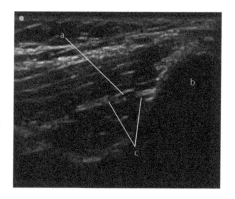

Genitofemoral block

COMPLEXITY: ⚫⚫⚫

Indications
- Herniorrhaphy, orchidopexy, or hydrocelectomy, in conjunction with ilioinguinal iliohypogastric block
- Long saphenous vein stripping, in addition to femoral nerve block
- Diagnosis of genitofemoral neuralgia.

See Figures 5.31 and 5.32.

Ultrasound-guided technique
Patient position: supine.

Landmarks: surface: pubic tubercle, inguinal ligament, inguinal crease, femoral artery.

Technique: identify the femoral artery. To block the femoral branch of the genitofemoral nerve, insert the needle at the lateral border of the femoral artery superior to the inguinal crease. Inject 2–5 mL of local anaesthetic under ultrasound guidance, just superficial to the femoral artery.

Needle: 25 G, 5 cm.

Local anaesthetic: 0.2% ropivacaine.

Comments: large-volume block at this level risks spread to the femoral nerve.

FIGURE 5.31 Insert the needle superior to the inguinal crease, using an IP approach.

a   Costal margin
b   ASIS
c   Right thigh
d   Inguinal crease

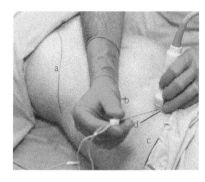

FIGURE 5.32
SAX view of the genitofemoral nerve.

a   Iliopectineal fascia
b   Femoral a.
c   Genitofemoral n.

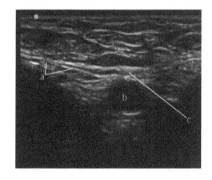

Dorsal penile block

COMPLEXITY: ⬤⬤⬤

Indications
- Dorsal slit of the foreskin
- Phimosis reduction
- Paraphimosis reduction
- Repair of penile lacerations.

See Figure 5.33 to 5.36.

Ultrasound-guided technique

Patient position: supine.

Landmarks: surface: base of the penis.

Technique: scan in transverse and sagittal planes to identify the base of the penis and suspensory ligaments; these structures define a triangular space. Insert the needle under ultrasound guidance 0.25 cm laterally to the suspensory ligament on either side, and fill the triangular space with 2–4 mL local anaesthetic.

Needle: 25 G, 1.5 cm.

Local anaesthetic: 0.75% ropivacaine.

FIGURE 5.33 Dorsal penile pre-block.

1   Penis
2   Urethra
3   Scrotum
4   Probe
5   Needle
6   Superficial fascia
7   Pubic symphysis
8   Triangular space where local anaesthetic is injected
9   Deep fascia
10 Dorsal nerve of the penis

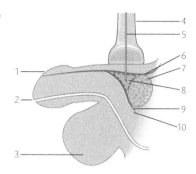

FIGURE 5.34 Transverse cross-section through the base of the penis.

1   Probe
2   Needle
3   Skin
4   Superficial fascia
5   Suspensory ligament
6   Dorsal nerve of penis
7   Penis
8   Urethra

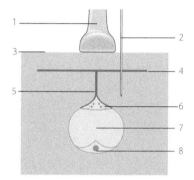

FIGURE 5.35 Dorsal penile pre-block.

a   Base of penis
b   Superficial fascia

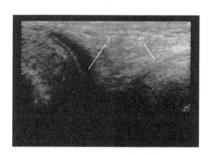

FIGURE 5.36 Dorsal penile post-block needle in situ.

a   Needle shaft
b   Triangular-shaped local anaesthetic expansion
c   Penis

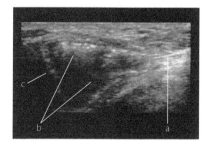

References

1 Vila HJ and Kavasmaneck D (2007). Paravertebral block: new benefits from an old procedure. *Curr Opin Anesthesiol* **20**, 316–18.
2 Hebbard P. *New 'sub-costal oblique' TAP block and audit data.* Parkville: HeartWeb. Viewed 7 September 2009, <http://www.heartweb.com.au/www/559/1001127/search.asp?frombox=true&searchstring=TAP+block&selecttype=3>.

INDEX

Management of severe local anaesthetic toxicity—quick reference safety guideline

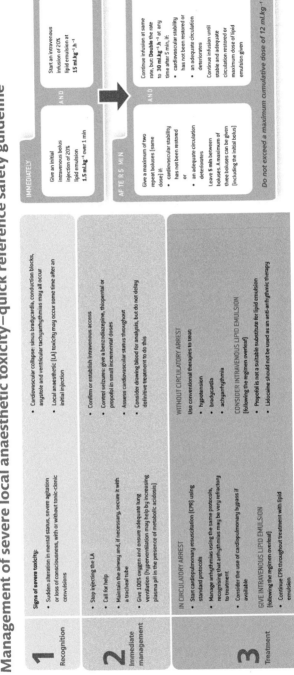

1 Recognition

Signs of severe toxicity:

- Sudden alteration in mental status, severe agitation or loss of consciousness, with or without tonic-clonic convulsions
- Cardiovascular collapse: sinus bradycardia, conduction blocks, asystole and ventricular tachyarrhythmias may all occur
- Local anaesthetic (LA) toxicity may occur some time after an initial injection

2 Immediate management

- Stop injecting the LA
- Call for help
- Maintain the airway and, if necessary, secure it with a tracheal tube
- Give 100% oxygen and ensure adequate lung ventilation (hyperventilation may help by increasing plasma pH in the presence of metabolic acidosis)
- Confirm or establish intravenous access
- Control seizures: give a benzodiazepine, thiopental or propofol in small incremental doses
- Assess cardiovascular status throughout
- Consider drawing blood for analysis, but do not delay definitive treatment to do this

3 Treatment

IN CIRCULATORY ARREST

- Start cardiopulmonary resuscitation (CPR) using standard protocols
- Manage arrhythmias using the same protocols, recognising that arrhythmias may be very refractory to treatment
- Consider the use of cardiopulmonary bypass if available

GIVE INTRAVENOUS LIPID EMULSION
[following the regimen overleaf]

- Continue CPR throughout treatment with lipid emulsion

WITHOUT CIRCULATORY ARREST

Use conventional therapies to treat:

- hypotension
- bradycardia
- tachyarrhythmia

CONSIDER INTRAVENOUS LIPID EMULSION
[following the regimen overleaf]

- Propofol is not a suitable substitute for lipid emulsion
- Lidocaine should not be used as an anti-arrhythmic therapy

IMMEDIATELY

Give an initial intravenous bolus injection of 20% lipid emulsion **1.5 mL.kg⁻¹ over 1 min**

AND

Start an intravenous infusion of 20% lipid emulsion at **15 mL.kg⁻¹.h⁻¹**

AFTER 5 MIN

Give a maximum of two repeat boluses [same dose] if:

- cardiovascular stability has not been restored

or

- an adequate circulation deteriorates

Leave 5 min between boluses. A maximum of three boluses can be given [including the initial bolus]

AND

Continue infusion at same rate, but: **Double the rate to 30 mL.kg⁻¹.h⁻¹** at any time after 5 min, if:

- cardiovascular stability has not been restored or
- an adequate circulation deteriorates

Continue infusion until stable and adequate circulation restored or maximum dose of lipid emulsion given

Do not exceed a maximum cumulative dose of 12 mL.kg⁻¹

- Recovery from LA-induced cardiac arrest may take >1 h
- Propofol is not a suitable substitute for lipid emulsion
- Lidocaine should not be used as an anti-arrhythmic therapy

4
Follow-up

- Arrange safe transfer to a clinical area with appropriate equipment and suitable staff until sustained recovery is achieved
- Exclude pancreatitis by regular clinical review, including daily amylase or lipase assays for two days

- Report cases to the appropriate organisation (eg. ANZCA). Please refer to their website for further information (www.anzca.edu.au)

  If Lipid has been given, please also report its use to the international registry at www.lipidregistry.org. Details may also be posted at (www.lipidrescue.org)

This AAGBI Safety Guideline was produced by a Working Party that comprised: Grant Cave, Will Harrop-Griffiths (Chair), Martyn Harvey, Tim Meek, John Picard, Tim Short and Guy Weinberg.

This Safety Guideline is endorsed by the Australian and New Zealand College of Anaesthetists (ANZCA).

© The Association of Anaesthetists of Great Britain & Ireland 2010

Your nearest bag of Lipid Emulsion is kept............................

An approximate dose regimen for a 70-kg patient would be as follows:

IMMEDIATELY

| Give an initial intravenous bolus injection of 20% lipid emulsion 100 ml over 1 min | AND | Start an intravenous infusion of 20% lipid emulsion at 1000 ml.h⁻¹ |

AFTER 5 MIN

| Give a maximum of two repeat boluses of 100 ml | AND | Continue infusion at same rate but **double** rate to 2000 ml.h⁻¹ if indicated at any time |

Do not exceed a maximum cumulative dose of 840 ml

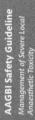

AAGBI Safety Guideline
Management of Severe Local Anaesthetic Toxicity